THE NATURAL WAY FOR DOGS AND CATS

The Natural Way for Dogs and Cats

Natural Treatments and Remedies for your Pet

MIDI FAIRGRIEVE

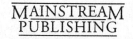
MAINSTREAM
PUBLISHING

EDINBURGH AND LONDON

First published in Great Britain in 1998 by
MAINSTREAM PUBLISHING COMPANY (EDINBURGH) LTD
7 Albany Street
Edinburgh EH1 3UG

ISBN 1 85158 973 2

A catalogue record for this book is available from the British Library

Typeset in Bembo
Printed and bound by WSOY, Finland

Contents

Acknowledgements

I would like to thank the following people for helping me with my research for this book and for giving their time and expertise freely and willingly: the Hon. Richard Arthur (McTimoney chiropractic), Christy Casley (healing), Keren Brynes (herbal medicine), Mary Boughton (herbal medicine), Sarah Fisher (aromatherapy and T-touch), Helen Gould (acupuncture), Dana Green (McTimoney chiropractic), Clare Harvey (flower essences), Daniel M. Iannarelli (osteopathy), Alasdair MacFarlane Govan (acupuncture), Christine Newman (Bach flower remedies), John A. Rohrbach (herbal medicine), June Third-Carter (homoeopathy) and The Self-Realisation Meditation Healing Centre, Somerset (healing).

I would also like to thank the following friends and family members for their enthusiasm and support throughout the writing of this book: Pat Agnew, Laura Borkovy, Alison De Marco and her pets, Aurora and Mr Pink (front cover), Rosie Filipiak and Steve Godfrey.

CHAPTER ONE

Introduction

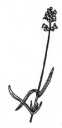

Nature has always held a cure for disease and it is only natural that we are returning to her for the answers, both for ourselves and for our animals. It is easy to forget that before modern medicine people and animals looked to nature for a cure. It is not surprising, then, that as more and more people are choosing natural treatments and remedies for themselves, they are also seeking them for their pets.

It is also becoming easier to find someone who will treat your pet holistically. More and more vets are combining complementary treatments with standard veterinary care or are willing to refer you to a natural therapist who works with animals. This growth in complementary medicine in the animal world is due partly to demand by pet owners for a more holistic practice of animal care and partly to the fact that vets themselves have found that modern drugs are not the only answer.

Many of the natural treatments detailed in this book have been around for hundreds, sometimes thousands, of years – which in itself is testimony to their curative powers. Animals have been treated by traditional means for as long as people have, and although complementary medicine may seem 'new', we are largely just rediscovering old systems of health care. Animals have always had an awareness of nature's medicinal powers and will look for edible plant cures in times of need.

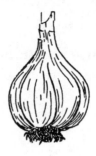

In practice, natural medicine works in an holistic way, which means it takes account of the animal's whole being (mind-body-spirit) and looks at all the different factors that are causing disease. In this way, treatment is directed at strengthening and supporting the total health of an animal and awakening its own powers of recovery. Rather than attacking the individual symptoms of disease, natural medicine aims to return the animal's mind, body and spirit to a balanced state so that the disease does not recur. This often involves permanent dietary and lifestyle changes for your pet. Without change, there can be no change!

'Mammalian bodies are designed to live a healthy life, and the body has a tendency to make efforts to return to being healthy. So when you are looking at things holistically you are attempting to help the body to return to being healthy. You are also trying to remove the influences – medicinal, nutritional or environmental – which are harmful and which lead to ill health.'
John A. Rohrbach, MVetMed, MRCVS

Both modern medicine and natural alternatives have a place in animal care. Sometimes drugs and surgery are the only ways to save an animal's life, particularly in accident and emergency situations. Drugs can also help to 'buy time' while the more slow-acting natural treatments take hold. The important thing is to respect the strengths and weaknesses of both forms of medicine and to use whichever is better for your pet. However, with less serious conditions, natural remedies support and strengthen the animal and do not have adverse side effects, which makes them a healthy alternative. Natural remedies are also inexpensive, safe to use at home and widely available.

The emphasis of natural medicine has always been on prevention. It stresses that by taking time to reassess your pet's diet and lifestyle, you can do a lot to improve their general health and reduce the chances of them becoming ill. Pets often mirror the state of mind of their owners, picking up on any negative emotions around them. For example, a pet living in a disharmonious household may well become ill or start to display behavioural problems as a result. Often the whole household needs to take the same remedy as their pet! There are also lots of factors that contribute to disease, including pollution of our water, air and soil, chemical fertilisers and pesticides in farming, the additions of synthetic flavourings and preservatives in food – the list is long! All these things put stress on the immune system and animals are just as vulnerable to these negative health factors as we are.

One of the main characteristics of health care in Western society is wanting instant answers and instant cures. In many ways we have become a quick-fix society, and this rubs off on to our pets. They get given instant meals day in, day out, and when they become ill, we do not consider that their diet and lifestyle might be the problem. Instead, we look for instant cures to heal them.

Many people want and expect miracle cures, but nature does not work like this. Natural medicine works with an animal's self-healing mechanism in a gentle way, bringing it back into balance and harmony. Always bear in mind the holistic nature of true healing and understand that disease is the result of a larger picture of lifestyle, diet and environmental factors. Giving natural remedies without changing other important factors may not cure your pet for long. The aim of this book is to encourage permanent healthy changes in your pet's life. For example, if your pet has cystitis you could use a homoeopathic remedy to clear it up – but it would be much better if you also changed the conditions that made it possible for the cystitis to occur in the first place. This might involve permanent changes in the diet including the regular addition of herbs, nutrients and natural remedies that support the urinary tract and the immune system in fighting infections. There may also be emotional factors at play which are weakening the animal's resistance to disease, and these can be healed with flower essences or healing. This is the true nature of holistic health care.

A good diet is at the core of a healthy life and is the foundation of successful treatment. We need to take responsibility for our pet's health and general well-being. All the treatments and remedies in this book will be enhanced by a natural preservative-free diet, and in many cases dietary changes alone can bring remarkable improvements in your pet's health. Many diseases suffered by cats and dogs these days can be avoided, including some of the chronic ones like heart disease, cancer and diabetes which have increased in line with our fast-food society.

The following chapters describe in detail the major holistic treatments for animals, how they work and what they can help. These include aromatherapy, acupuncture, biochemical tissue salts, chiropractic, diet and food supplements, flower essences, healing, herbs, homoeopathy, osteopathy, and T-touch. Each chapter also tells you how to contact someone who can treat your pet and, where relevant, how to put together a natural remedies medicine chest for use at home.

Chapters 15 and 16 list specific ailments and conditions and include suggested remedies and details of first-aid treatments. Whichever remedies and treatments you decide to use, make sure you read the relevant chapters to get an understanding of what that treatment involves. This is especially important when carrying out the treatment yourself. Natural remedies are not meant to replace veterinary care for a seriously ill pet; however, many vets also practise complementary treatments, and those who do not are often happy to refer you to somebody who does. When opting for natural treatments and remedies, keep your vet informed of what you are doing.

Remember, prevention is better than cure.

CHAPTER TWO

Ten Tips to Keep your Pet Happy and Healthy

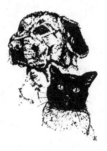

Your pets need ...

1. Fresh air, sunshine and regular exercise. Dogs enjoy running around and sniffing out new smells, or just lying in the sun on a warm day. Cats are night-time creatures and love being outside at night, when they can hunt and prowl.

2. A healthy diet. A natural preservative-free diet is the best diet you can give your pet. They need fresh water every day, preferably filtered or bottled mineral water. Do not give snacks between meals because it encourages animals to hang around constantly expecting food – which can become irritating for you and makes them unable to settle.

3. Clear boundaries and adequate discipline. Pets need to know what they can and cannot do: which parts of the

house or furniture they can use, what they can chew and what they cannot chew, and so on. Cats (especially ones that do not get out that much) need a scratching post, or you may find your furniture serving the same purpose!

4. Their own bed, which should be warm and comfortable and made of natural fibres. Old wool blankets can be picked up cheaply in charity shops and make great bedding material. Just like us, our pets sometimes want to have peace and quiet and need to have a place that is just for them. They also need enough rest.

5. Love and attention, companionship, touch. Most pets enjoy being touched by their owners, and it is therapeutic for them. It also shows them that you love them, which makes for a contented animal.

6. Regular grooming and occasional bathing for dogs. Cats are good groomers and rarely need a wash. Most dogs love to play in water, so take them to places they can splash about and swim.

7. Play, such as chasing sticks, playing with toys, socialising with other animals. Animals enjoy interacting with their own kind and learning their own social hierarchy.

8. A job to do. This refers mainly to dogs. Some breeds are workers and need to be occupied doing jobs such as guarding, herding and racing. Bored animals can become disturbed and difficult

9. Routine. Animals like a routine which they can rely on.

10. To be treated as an animal, not as a human being!

CHAPTER THREE

A Healthy Diet

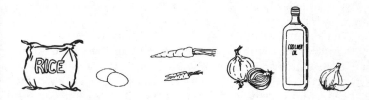

All healing begins with optimum nutrition

A healthy diet is the key to a healthy pet – which is why diet and food supplements are the first two subjects covered by this book. They are the most important contributions you can make to your pet's health – after all, feeding is the one thing you are able to influence for better or for worse. Animals on a preservative-free, natural diet rarely become ill because their bodies are better able to resist disease. The ultimate success of all of the treatments and remedies in the following chapters depends on a good diet.

Whatsoever was the Father of a disease, an ill diet was the Mother
– Chinese Proverb

Just what is a healthy diet for dogs and cats? We are bombarded with so much information these days that it has become very confusing to know what is best for our pets. Is dried food better than tinned food? And what about the semi-moist foods, maybe they are better? Many people are scared not to buy commercially prepared 'complete' or 'balanced' foods in case they get it wrong and cause malnutrition in their pets. However, imagine bringing up a child solely on 'convenience foods' and expecting them to become a healthy, vibrant adult. We all know that fresh food is vital for good health, and that includes eating some of it raw. Commercially prepared pet foods are more or less 'convenience foods for pets', and most cats and dogs are fed tinned or dried food throughout their entire life.

A lot of health problems are food-orientated, and you can do so much for your pet by making a few simple changes to their daily diet. Don't be scared to make your own pet food. Cats and dogs have specific requirements, but if you follow the advice given in this book on diet and supplements your pet will be a lot healthier in the long run.

Nutrition is the pivot upon which health and disease balance

Just as the number of people suffering from chronic diseases such as arthritis, cancer, allergies, obesity, heart disease, skin problems and diabetes is on the increase, so is the number of pets suffering similar problems. This increase of ill health goes hand in hand with the increase of processed and refined foods in the diet of both pets and people. In the case of your pet, some of the early warning signs of a poor-quality diet are a dull or smelly coat, skin problems, scratching, excess moulting, weight problems, bad breath, diarrhoea and constipation.

Good-quality food for your dog or cat is the key to preventative health and is a vital factor in recovery. Whatever natural treatments or remedies you use, they will always be enhanced by a healthy, well-balanced diet. In fact, changing your pet's diet alone can produce spectacular improvements in their health and help them to avoid disease in the first place. A healthy diet has a big impact on an animal's energy levels, appearance, performance and general health. This means making your pet's food from scratch, using fresh, wholesome ingredients with additional supplements. This is the best way to ensure a happy and healthy life.

The effects of a change of diet can be quite astonishing. Your pet may at last be free of a smelly skin, digestive problems, arthritis, obesity, behavioural problems and allergies. This is because a healthy, natural diet promotes the elimination of waste, reduces the intake of harmful substances and increases an animal's resistance to disease.

Commercially prepared pet food

Pet food sits at the bottom of the pile as far as quality is concerned, and as food generally becomes less healthy, our pets are bearing the brunt. Ready-made pet foods vary in quality and nutritional value. While some are well-balanced and made from relatively good ingredients, others contain poor-quality ingredients and a host of harmful preservatives and additives. However, the exclusive use of commercially prepared pet food, whatever the quality, with no additional fresh food, makes for an unbalanced and unhealthy diet.

Dogs and cats often smell like the food they eat – if it isn't nice then it's time to change their diet!

What to watch out for

TINNED FOOD

Most tinned cat and dog food contain meat which may be labelled as 'meat derivatives' or 'meat by-products'. This is often low quality and includes ears, horns, hooves, hides, beaks, feathers, entrails, high amounts of saturated fats, and diseased meat that has been passed unfit for human consumption. The problem with poor-quality protein is that it increases the workload for the liver and kidneys. Animals need high-quality protein, like muscle meat, eggs and fish. Tinned food may also contain vegetable protein derived from cereals, texturised vegetable protein and soya, much of which is waste by-products of the human food industry, and again of suspect quality.

DRIED FOODS

Dried foods have become increasingly popular because they are so convenient. You just open the packet, pour the right amount into the pet's bowl and that's that – no variety, no fresh meat, no fresh vegetables and often inadequate nutrition in the long term.

Apart from the above, dried foods are the subject of much controversy because they absorb so much fluid from the animal's digestive tract. Although dried-food manufacturers always recommend ensuring plenty of fresh water is available, you cannot be certain your pet will drink extra water to compensate. Try soaking some dried food overnight and see just how much water it takes up! If you do use a dried food, always soak it for at least half an hour to ensure your pet gets enough fluid. If they are not getting enough water to flush out metabolic wastes, then kidney problems can result. Dried foods are also thought to contribute to kidney problems and cystitis due to their poor-quality protein content which upsets the body's acid/alkaline balance.

Poor-quality dried foods also have many of the negative factors associated with the meat and vegetable protein content of tinned foods, as well as a host of unhealthy additives and preservatives – with growing concern especially over the 'permitted' antioxidants. Reports from America suggest that some antioxidants may be related to a number of health problems, namely liver cancer, skin allergies, auto-immune diseases and reproductive problems. Chronic disease in our pets has been increasing in line with the use of commercially prepared pet foods.

SEMI-MOIST FOODS
The main problem with these is the amount of sugar they contain, in some cases up to 25 per cent! Animals can get addicted to sugar and become really picky about eating anything else. Sugar is a bringer of disease, sooner or later, including diabetes, allergies, cataracts, obesity, nervousness and tooth decay. Have you ever wondered how the semi-moist foods can last so long without needing to be kept in the fridge? Well, you've guessed it – the high sugar content acts as a preservative.

ADDITIVES
Most commercially made pet foods contain a host of additives, colourings, flavourings and preservatives, high quantities of sugar and salt, and other contaminants like antibiotic and growth-hormone residues from meat, heavy metals and agricultural chemical and pesticide residues. Toxins gather in the tissues and it is thought that the accumulative toxic effect of these can lead to all sorts of health problems, including liver and kidney disease, cancer, lowered immunity, skin problems, hair loss and behavioural problems, such as anxiety and aggression. High amounts of salt can lead to heart disease and kidney failure. High amounts of sugar can lead to diabetes, obesity, heart trouble and a long list of other health problems.

Commercially prepared pet foods are often heat-treated, which destroys a lot of the naturally occurring vitamins and enzymes. They also contain some of the primary allergens as their main ingredient – beef, wheat, dairy produce, corn, tuna fish and soya – which puts further stress on an animal's health.

Lead and other heavy metals contaminate pet foods as a result of processing and canning. They adversely affect the immune system and leave animals open to disease. In America, the American Medical Association reported that people who ate cat and dog food were in danger of consuming toxic levels of lead! Tuna fish is often contaminated with high amounts of mercury and should therefore be avoided.

Are all ready-made pet foods inadequate?

If you do have to use a ready-made pet food, buy one that is labelled free of unwanted elements. Look out for the following foods and try to avoid them: wheat, wheat gluten, dairy produce, soya, cheap bulking agents, cereals, beef, pork, artificial flavourings, colourings, preservatives, taste enhancers, added salt, sugar, meat by-products and meat derivatives.

The better-quality pet foods have the advantage of being free of the main food allergens. They tend to be made from brown rice, millet, lamb and poultry, and not from meat 'by-products' and 'substandard' grains. They also contain good-quality fats. This type of food is the next best thing to making it yourself, as it is relatively clean, wholesome and well-balanced. Some of the brand names to look out for include Denes, Burns, James Wellbeloved, Omega and Butchers.

Although a natural preservative-free diet is the best diet you can give to your pet, there are times when a ready-made pet food makes life easier, such as if you are going away for the weekend or leaving your pet with somebody else for short periods of time. However, it is best to make their diet from scratch whenever possible and leave the convenience foods for emergencies. It is a question of doing the best that you can and getting into new ways and habits of preparing pet food.

Some dos and don'ts when using ready-prepared pet foods

- Never just use tinned meat. Always add a cooked grain or dry biscuit meal to your pet's daily diet.

- Do not feed cats with dog food, since cats need a higher protein content in their food than dogs.

- Dried food needs to be soaked in water for at least an hour.

- Dried 'complete' foods often need to have oils added to them: a mixture of vegetable oils, fish and fish liver oils, meat fat, dripping, etc. Use one teaspoon daily for cats, and up to one tablespoon daily for dogs, depending on their size.

- Commercially prepared dog and cat foods often need to have food supplements added to ensure optimum health, especially when an animal is recovering from illness or at times of increased need, such as pregnancy (see chapter four).

- Always read labels and know what is in the food you are buying. Avoid regularly using pet foods containing harmful ingredients (see previous page).

What is a healthy diet for cats and dogs?

Cats and dogs are meat-eating animals (carnivores) and therefore need to be treated as such. Just because you may prefer to be vegetarian, it does not mean that it is healthier for your pet. In fact, you can seriously damage animals' health by not feeding them meat, especially cats. Dogs are by nature omnivorous, so it is easier to feed them a variety of foods – even fruit, if they like it – but they still need a proportion of good-quality meat in their diet.

A well-balanced, fresh, wholesome, preservative-free homemade diet is simple to prepare and often works out cheaper than ready-made pet foods. The main ingredients of a daily diet should include protein, fat, carbohydrate, vegetables (and occasionally fruit, if they like it) and food supplements. The meat and vegetables are best served raw or lightly cooked; grains need to be cooked. Fats should be a mixture of saturated (hard fats) and unsaturated (oils). This type of diet is close to what your pet would eat in the wild. It is always better for your pet's health to use organic ingredients where possible.

PROTEIN
Cats and dogs are carnivorous animals and need to be given meat as

their main source of protein. Other sources of good-quality protein include fish, eggs, cottage cheese and live yoghurt. Vegetable protein (lentils, beans, tofu, etc.) can be fed to dogs as long as it is combined with a grain to make the protein content complete. Some people feel that a dog can be fed quite adequately on a vegetarian diet; however, this does need to be done with rigorous attention to the principles of vegetarianism and supplements are essential. The protein content of a cat's diet should be about 35–40 per cent, and for a dog the content should be about 25–30 per cent. This means that including the fat content of meat (or other protein source), about 60 per cent of a cat's diet should be meat, and 35–40 per cent of a dog's diet.

Meat Most meat is best served raw (or cooked as little as possible) since there is great nutritional value in raw meat, including digestive enzymes and vitamins which can be destroyed by cooking. Cats must have meat protein in order to get sufficient amounts of the amino acid taurine, which is only found in meat. You can buy fresh raw meat from your local butcher. The cheaper cuts are fine for pets, and try to include some offal once or twice a week: hearts, kidney, liver, lung or tripe. This can be cut up into bite-size pieces and given raw. Offal adds valuable trace minerals and vitamins to the diet. Cats enjoy chicken necks. Your butcher may be prepared to mince the chicken necks and gizzards for you or you can mince your own meat at home. Pork should always be cooked.

Raw minced meat for cats and dogs is widely available from kennels, pet shops and most of the big pet superstores. It comes frozen and guaranteed free of cereals, additives, preservatives, colourings, heads, feet and other low-grade animal parts. The range of meat available includes chicken, turkey, tripe, lamb, beef, rabbit and fish and works out cheaper than tinned meat and is also of a human food standard and is a high-quality source of protein.

Fish Dogs and cats like fish, but be aware that it can be an allergy trigger. If you suspect an allergy to fish, then leave it out. Raw, frozen, minced fish can be bought from pet shops, kennels and pet superstores, or you can buy it fresh and use it raw or lightly cooked. Tinned fish such as sardines, mackerel and pilchards can occasionally be used. Fish heads and tails make great stock and you can cook grains in it for extra flavour.

Eggs Eggs are a high-quality protein and can be added regularly to your pet's diet, but try to use organic or free-range eggs.

Dairy produce Not all animals can digest milk; it is therefore best to avoid it. Yoghurt, cottage cheese and goat's milk are exceptions to this and can form some of the protein element of the diet. Unpasteurised milk is also acceptable in small amounts.

Vegetable protein Vegetable protein can play a small part in your pet's diet, although you must make sure it is always combined with a grain in order to make the protein content complete. Cats really should get all their protein from meat, but dogs can have some protein from vegetable sources, e.g. beans, lentils, soya mince and tofu.

FATS AND OILS
Dogs and cats need saturated fats (animal fats) as well as unsaturated fats (vegetable and fish oils). The fat content of a cat's diet should be about 25–30 per cent, and fat should make up about 15–20 per cent of a dog's diet. (Much of this may well be included in the meat proportion of the diet.) Don't make the mistake of cutting saturated fats out of your pet's diet because you think it is better for their health; they do need some, especially cats. Fats are essential to a healthy body and a glossy coat. Leftover bacon fat from cooking is a great way to add fat and flavour to your pet's food; other saturated fats include butter, beef dripping and meat fat. Oils in the diet include fish and fish liver oil, and vegetable oils such as corn, sunflower, olive or linseed. A daily dose of vegetable oil helps to prevent fur balls in cats. Vegetable proteins and organ meats have less fat than muscle meat, so you may have to bump up the fat content of the diet when using these. Most skin and coat problems indicate a lack of essential fats in the diet.

CARBOHYDRATES
These provide energy and should make up about 60 per cent of a dog's diet and about 40 per cent of a cat's diet.

Grains Fresh, whole, unrefined grains including brown rice, millet, oats, barley and buckwheat are the best source of carbohydrate and need to be included in the diet every day. All grains have to be cooked to open the starch granules so that they are more easily digested, but you can cook a fews days' worth at a time and keep it in the fridge. The single most important grain is brown rice, and this can be the staple carbohydrate of your pet's diet with other grains

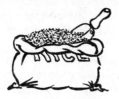

added for variety. Because many of these whole grains take a while to cook, one of the easiest ways to cook them is to bring the pan to the boil, simmer for ten minutes, then turn off the heat. As long as the lid is tightly fitting, the grain will have soaked up the water and be fully cooked by the time it has cooled.

All of the above grains are just as nutritious as wheat, but do not cause the allergic problems associated with wheat. If you can get organic grains, this is always preferable. Oats contain iron and help cleanse the intestine; barley is a blood cleanser and a good remedy for kidney and bladder problems.

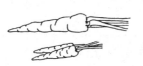

Vegetables These are an important addition to your pet's diet and can be given lightly cooked or raw. In the wild, cats and dogs would have got much of their vegetable food from eating the stomach contents of their prey, which would provide them with important minerals and vitamins. Collect up leftover vegetables or the bits you might normally throw away, like potato peelings, the outside leaves of cabbage and lettuce, broccoli stalks and cauliflower leaves, and finely chop them up (food processors are good for this) and add them to your pet's meal. Cats will eat vegetables if they are chopped up small enough and mixed with something tasty. You can also cook potato peelings and vegetable ends in with the grains. Root vegetables, like carrots, parsnips and beetroot, are best grated and added raw. Some vegetables have specific healing effects and can be added to your pet's diet depending on what is needed. Onions and garlic, for example, cleanse the blood and prevent worms. Raw sprouted seeds are also highly nutritious and are vital foods.

Fruit If your pet likes fruit then it makes a healthy treat, used instead of the highly coloured and flavoured pet treats that are available. Fresh or dried fruit can be given, although dogs tend to like fruit more than cats. My own dog will happily eat a whole pear and will take them off the tree himself. My sister's dogs readily eat windfall apples and will 'climb' the plum trees to get at the ripe plums! Fruit, like vegetables, have specific therapeutic powers and can be added to the diet as necessary. You may have to cut fruit up really finely for cats and mix it in with their meal rather than feeding it to them separately. Citrus fruits are not recommended as they are generally too acid for dogs and cats.

Fruit and vegetables also make a great treat or snack and many pets will be just as happy with a raw carrot or a piece of apple as they would with a less healthy alternative.

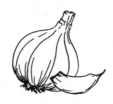

HERBS
Culinary herbs, such as parsley, sage, mint, basil, lovage, thyme, oregano, marjoram and savory, and garlic can be added regularly to pet food. Animals will instinctively seek out herbs to eat in the wild. These can be used fresh or dried.

BONES
Raw bones are also an important element in your pet's diet since they exercise the teeth and jaws and provide essential minerals,

particularly calcium which balances the high phosphorus content of meat. Raw bones also act like a natural toothbrush and keep your pet's teeth healthy and clean. The best ones for dogs are marrow bones, but never poultry or other fine bones as they can splinter too easily. Cats can be given chicken necks and wings to chew on. Do not give either cats or dogs pork bones or fish bones. If your pet does not get bones, make sure you add bonemeal or a calcium supplement occasionally to their diet. Cooked bones are fine for indoor toys as long as your pet is also getting raw bones.

LEFTOVERS

Leftover food can be collected up and given to your pet at their next meal. Meaty leftovers are great for cats, and dogs will finish up almost any kind of food such as salad, vegetables, meaty scraps or baked potato skins. Do not give them the unhealthy leftovers like puddings, pastries and sugary food, though!

RAW FOOD VERSUS COOKED FOOD

Raw food is important because it contains many important elements that can be lost or destroyed by cooking, such as digestive enzymes and vitamins and minerals. Raw food is also 'alive' in that it is filled with life force energy vital for good health, and this reason alone makes it important to feed your pet some food raw. Grains need to be cooked to make them digestible, but meat and vegetables have much more value when eaten raw.

Changing to a new diet

It can take time to change to a new way of feeding your pet and to get into different routines when cooking and shopping. It can also take time for them to get used to new tastes and textures, especially if they have been used to diets high in sugars and salts. Some animals can become addicted to some of the commercially prepared foods and to tuna fish (which can also have a dangerously high mercury content). Just persevere until you succeed. Sometimes fasting a healthy animal for a day or two helps to heighten their hunger for new and different foods and break a habit of finicky eating! One of the best ways of changing their diet is to introduce the new food gradually and phase out the old food at the same time. You might want to do this over a week or two.

Make it fun!

Cooking for your pet need not be a chore and it is fun to try new recipes now and again. One of the best books for recipe ideas is *The Healthy Cat and Dog Cookbook* by Joan Harper (see end of chapter for details). As your pet's health improves, you may find yourself following some of the same healthy principles!

How many meals a day?

A healthy cat or dog in general only needs one meal per day, although puppies, kittens and older pets will need to have several small meals spread throughout the day. There are no hard and fast rules about when is the best time to feed your pet, and usually you will find a time that suits you and your pet. The most important thing is that meal times are regular.

How much food?

Animals differ in their needs, so the best way to work out how much food your pet needs is to use a commonsense approach – if they gain weight, then cut down on their food; and if they lose weight, add more. So much depends on their daily activity, age, breed and other individual influences. Excessive weight gain or weight loss could be a sign of a serious illness, and in this case it would be advisable to take your pet to the vet.

Elderly pets, puppies and kittens will have different nutritional needs. This will be covered later in the book.

Allergies

Allergies and allergy-based diseases are becoming more frequent in pets and inadequate diet is thought to be one of the main contributing factors. Symptoms of allergy can be many and varied, but some common ones include sneezing, scratching, fur loss, reactions to flea bites, diarrhoea and constipation. Behavioural problems too are associated with allergies – just like children, pets are sensitive to E numbers! Colourings are not put in food for an animal's benefit and are totally unnecessary. Allergic reactions can be caused by environmental elements too, like house dust, dust mites and pollens. A poor or inadequate diet impairs the digestive system and damages the immune system to the extent that it cannot function properly and becomes oversensitive.

Common trigger foods

These include beef, pork, milk products, corn, wheat and wheat gluten, eggs, soya, yeast and tuna fish.

Commercially prepared foods use some of the primary allergens as their main ingredients. The damaging effects will be much worse if these foods are also full of artificial dyes, preservatives, sugar, salt and flavourings.

What do I feed an allergic pet?

First cut out all the possible allergens from their diet and environment. A one-day fast is helpful in clearing the system of toxins (see fasting), and then reintroduce food starting with foods that are not usually a problem, like brown rice and lamb. Raw carrots can also be added to their meal along with fats and oils. Stick to this for at least a week with no other type of food and see if your pet's symptoms and general health improves. After a week you can begin to reintroduce new foods one day at a time and watch to see if they cause any adverse reactions. If not, you can be fairly sure that your pet can tolerate that new food and it can become part of the whole diet. Any food that does cause an adverse reaction should be omitted.

When allergies are suspected, it is best to use bottled or filtered water only.

Supplements for an allergic pet

The most likely allergic trigger is brewer's yeast, or a yeast-based B vitamin or multi-vitamin complex. If yeast is a problem, look for yeast-free supplements. Many of the cat and dog multi-minerals and vitamins are also free of other possible allergenic substances such as dairy products, sugar, soya, gluten, corn, wheat, egg, artificial colourings and flavourings, so look out for these. Whether your pet is allergic or not, it is always better to use the better-quality supplements. Adding digestive enzymes to meals helps in cases of allergy. See chapter four for supplementing your pet's diet.

Feeding an elderly pet

Older pets have different dietary needs from younger animals. As dogs and cats grow older, their bodily functions can become less efficient, particularly when it comes to digesting food and eliminating waste products. They are also prone to putting on weight as they become less active. If your pet is gaining weight, reduce their food intake until you reach the optimum dietary amount for them.

An elderly pet's diet needs to be easy to digest and made up of good-quality ingredients.

The protein content of the diet of both cats and dogs should be moderately reduced to lessen the eliminative load on the kidneys, but make sure it is high-quality protein.

Add plenty of fibre such as brown rice, raw vegetables and psyllium husks, in order to avoid constipation.

Many older pets also need digestive enzymes and other dietary supplements to be added regularly to their food to ensure optimum nutrition (see chapter four).

To help with digestion, feed elderly pets on a little-and-often basis, rather than just one large meal in a day.

Feeding puppies and kittens

The healthier a young animal's diet is when they are growing, the better their overall health will be throughout their life. After weaning, a natural preservative-free diet is the best start you can give any young pet, and it helps to reduce the risk of allergies and behavioural problems arising. A good diet will help the immune system to grow strong and will protect your pet from disease.

The first six months are a time of rapid growth, and puppies and kittens will need twice as much food as their parents. They will also need to be fed at least three times a day. Puppies and kittens need a slightly higher percentage of protein and fat in their diet than adult dogs and cats. The diet can be enriched with egg yolks, honey, molasses, cod liver oil, brewer's yeast, vitamin C and bonemeal. Raw garlic or garlic capsules added to their food daily will help protect them from worms and other parasites (see chapter four for food supplements).

After six months, they only need to be fed twice a day, and then just once a day after nine months.

Make sure your puppy's diet is easy to digest and made from good-quality ingredients, especially good-quality protein and fat. It is always best to prepare their food from scratch using raw meat and cooked grains as the basis of the diet.

Always make sure your pet has fresh water available at all times.

Homemade treats for dogs and cats

Dog/Cat biscuits

2 tablespoons bran/bran flakes (e.g. wheat, oat or rye)

2 cups wholemeal flour (e.g. wheat, rice, rye, etc.)

1 heaped tablespoon crushed vitamin B complex tablets
(or brewer's yeast if no allergy is suspected)

1 cup wheat germ

2 teaspoons blackstrap molasses (1 teaspoon for cats)

1 tablespoon linseed oil or corn oil

1 oz butter (cats only)

1 teaspoon anchovy paste/fish paste (cats only)

Water

Mix all the ingredients together in a bowl and add enough water to
make a firm dough. Shape the dough into small, flat biscuit shapes and
bake in a moderate oven for about half an hour or until dry and hard.
The biscuits will keep for at least a week if stored in a cool, dry, airtight
container. All the above ingredients can be bought in health-food
shops. Linseed oil and molasses can also be bought in pet superstores
(usually in the horse-feed section). Substitute wheat bran and wheat
flour for an alternative grain if you suspect an allergy to wheat.

These make a really healthy treat and dogs seem to love them. They
also make a fun Christmas treat for children to make for their pets.

An ill pet
Never force an ill animal to eat; dogs and cats will naturally fast when
they are feeling unwell. Always make sure that plenty of fresh water
is available.

Fasting

Fasting is one of the best ways of detoxifying the body and stimulating healing. When energy is not being used up on digestive processes, the body can concentrate on repair, renewal and fighting disease. Fasting is particularly effective in healing infections, fevers, skin problems and digestive disorders. Animals in the wild will naturally fast when they are ill, and so will many domestic pets. Regular fasting of healthy animals will bring enormous health benefits and help to boost their immune systems and keep their bodies free of harmful toxins. Some animals do this naturally on a weekly basis, and you may wish to try introducing regular short fasts.

Fasting dos and don'ts

- Never fast a pet that is young, old, pregnant, lactating or ill, without veterinary supervision. Healthy mature pets can fast for a full day on a regular basis, but no more than one day a week.

- During a fast you can give your pet liquid nourishment such as:

  > Homemade barley water, with or without honey added to it. This is rich in magnesium and helps ease rheumatism and skin complaints, and it also purifies the blood. Simmer one tablespoon of pearl barley in fresh water for 20 minutes, cool and strain.

  > Homemade rice water. Simmer one tablespoon of brown rice in water for 40 minutes, strain and cool. You can add a few fenugreek seeds for added (curry) flavour.

  > Vegetable or chicken broth (the strained liquid only). Use a mixture of root vegetables, onions, garlic potato peelings and/or chicken bones simmered in water.

> Water and apple cider vinegar (plus honey if desired)
>
> Fish head broth (strained liquid only)
>
> Stock made from meat bones (strained liquid only)
>
> Aloe vera juice diluted with water – a wonderful detoxifier

- Dogs and cats can also be given bones on a fast day.

- Leave out any additional vitamins and minerals while fasting.

- Make sure your pet gets plenty of fresh air and light exercise.

- Give them lots of affection during a fast so they don't feel you have just forgotten to feed them!

- It is a good time to give them a bath with a natural herbal shampoo, especially if they have skin or coat problems.

- End the fast slowly with a small meal of wholesome ingredients.

When an ill animal does want food again, one of the most beneficial things you can do is to change their diet to a natural, homemade, preservative-free one plus supplements.

Feeding dos and don'ts

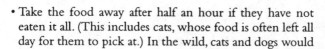

- Feed at the same time every day.

- Take the food away after half an hour if they have not eaten it all. (This includes cats, whose food is often left all day for them to pick at.) In the wild, cats and dogs would not have a constant source of food to pick at throughout the day and short periods of fasting between meals are very important for efficient detoxification.

• Fresh water should be available at all times, preferably filtered or mineral water.

• Do not feed from the table or give too many treats.

• Food and water bowls should be made of glass, stainless steel or porcelain.

• Cook food in stainless steel pans, not aluminium pans.

Useful information

Further reading
Reigning Cats and Dogs by Pat McKay; Oscar Publications
The New Natural Cat by Anitra Frazier; Plume Books
The Healthy Cat and Dog Cookbook by Joan Harper; Pet Press
Dr Pitcairn's Complete Guide to Natural Health for Cats and Dogs by Richard Pitcairn and Susan Hubble Pitcairn; Rodale Press
Natural Healing for Cats and Dogs by Diane Stein; The Crossing Press
Keep your Pet Healthy the Natural Way by Pat Lazarus; Keats Publishing

CHAPTER FOUR

Food Supplements

The question of whether supplements are necessary when the diet is 'balanced' or 'complete' is a much-debated point. Perhaps there would not be a need for supplements if our food contained everything that we and our pets need, but often this is not the case. Modern farming methods and the use of chemicals deplete the soil of essential nutrients and consequently our food is depleted. Food processing destroys valuable nutrients and enzymes. Synthetic additives and preservatives also increase the need for vitamins and minerals.

All animals are different, and each has individual needs. Some may need extra supplements every day, particularly if they work or exercise hard, whilst others may only need extra supplements in times of special need like illness, pregnancy, lactation, growth and old age. However, by adding food supplements on a regular basis to your pet's diet, you will improve their health and protect them from disease.

Vitamins, minerals and other essential nutrients can be powerful tools in curing disease.

Vitamins
Vitamins are vital to health and regulate body processes. They are easily destroyed by cooking and food processing, and therefore may need to be added to the diet despite claims of food being 'complete' or 'balanced'.

Vitamin A is vital for healthy eyes and good eyesight, and is important for maintaining strong bones and healthy skin, coat, teeth and gums. Vitamin A is also a powerful antioxidant which protects the body's cells and tissues from pollution damage and cancer. It also has immune-system-enhancing properties, and is particularly good for healing respiratory problems. It is vital for the development and growth of kittens and puppies. Too much vitamin A can be toxic, so it is always best to use food sources of vitamin A or supplement it as part of a balanced vitamin complex.

Good sources? Fish liver oil, liver and eggs. Vitamin A can be added to the diet as part of a multi-vitamin complex or added in a food source. The easiest way to supplement vitamin A is by adding fish liver oil to the diet.

How much? 400iu vitamin A weekly for cats, up to 3,000iu weekly for dogs, depending on size. Up to one teaspoon of fish liver oil weekly for cats, up to three teaspoons weekly for dogs. If you are already giving a multi-vitamin complex, beware of overdosing with vitamin A by adding liver or fish liver oil to the diet as well. Remember that animal liver is also high in vitamin A.

The B vitamins are essential for healthy organs and nervous system, glossy coat and healthy skin. Some of the B vitamins are needed for red-blood-cell formation. They help to keep parasites at bay, protect your pet from stress and boost the immune system. B vitamins are unlikely to be overdosed since they are water-soluble and any excess is naturally eliminated by the body.

Good sources? Whole grains, meat, eggs and brewer's yeast, or you can use a yeast-free vitamin B complex if your pet is allergic to yeast.

How much? Up to ½ a teaspoon brewer's yeast daily for cats, up to one tablespoon daily for dogs, sprinkled on their food. Cats and dogs generally love the taste of brewer's yeast. If they do have an allergy to yeast, buy a yeast-free vitamin B complex and reduce the human recommended amount to suit the size of your pet.

Although dogs and cats can make their own **vitamin C**, if their diet is inadequate or their health impaired then their ability to make adequate amounts of vitamin will also be impaired. Pet foods do not contain additional vitamin C because it is thought that dogs and cats can make enough in their bodies. It has been found to be a preventive against hip dysplasia, lameness, arthritis, viral diseases and skin problems.

Vitamin C is vital for healing cuts and wounds and internally damaged tissues, a healthy immune system, protecting against infection and cancer, and encouraging healthy skin, bones, cartilage, teeth and gums. It is also a major detoxifier, including heavy metals. A sick animal will have a great need for vitamin C and can be given large quantities up to the point of bowel tolerance. This is the point at which too much vitamin C will cause diarrhoea, but it is a very good guide to how much your pet's body needs.

Good sources? Green leafy vegetables, potatoes, cauliflower, nettles, parsley. Vitamin C powder can be sprinkled into food.

How much? On a daily basis, cats can have up to 500mg and dogs 500–7,000mg, depending on their size. See specific ailments for times of increased need such as illness, infections and wound healing.

Vitamin D is needed for the absorption of other nutrients such as calcium and phosphorus and is therefore essential in helping to maintain bone structure and healthy teeth. Like vitamin A, vitamin D can be toxic in large doses.

Good sources? Eggs, oily fish, sunlight. Fish liver oil is a good way to supplement both vitamin A and vitamin D. Reduce the amount of vitamin D during the summer months, when animals are getting more sunlight.

How much? 400iu weekly for cats, up to 10,000iu weekly for dogs. The best way to supplement vitamin D is with fish liver oil (¼–½) teaspoon for cats, ½–1 teaspoon for dogs, once or twice a week or as part of a multi-vitamin complex.

Vitamin E is a potent antioxidant which protects animals against pollution damage and cancer. Vitamin E enhances the effect of vitamin A. It also plays an important role in a healthy reproductive system and efficient lactation, a healthy heart and good circulation. It aids wound healing and can be used externally to promote skin healing. It also prevents fats from going rancid. Rancid fats are one of the worst known cancer-causing agents.

Good sources? Wheat germ oil, wheat germ, vegetable oils, whole grains, leafy greens. Vitamin E is also available in capsule form, but make sure you get a natural form of vitamin E and not a synthetic one. (For example, D-alpha tocopherol is a natural vitamin E, but a Dl prefix is not.)

How much? Up to 50–100iu daily for cats, up to 400iu daily for dogs, depending on their size.

Multi-vitamins are a simple and practical way of ensuring that your pet is getting a basic level of these essential nutrients. There are many good-quality ones available which are designed for cats and dogs and appropriately balanced for their different needs, such as Denes and The Missing Link (see 'Where to buy food supplements' at the end of the chapter). Most cat and dog multi-vitamins will need additional amounts of vitamins C and E added. A sick pet will need large quantities of vitamin C, up to bowel-tolerance levels.

A combination of fish liver oil, wheat germ oil, brewer's yeast, alfalfa and vitamin C powder will deliver all of the above vitamins and can replace the need for a multi-vitamin complex (see 'Other valuable supplements', page 38).

Minerals

Minerals are important for growth and development but they are often deficient in a pet's diet. Some minerals like calcium and magnesium are needed in large quantities, while others, such as zinc and selenium, are just needed in tiny amounts.

Calcium is essential for healthy bones and teeth as well as for keeping the nerves, heart and muscles healthy. Growing puppies and kittens, pregnant females and lactating mothers have a special need for calcium in the diet. Phosphorus (found in meat) can deplete calcium in the body; therefore, a diet too high in meat can cause calcium deficiency.
Good sources? Bonemeal, bones, sardines, green leafy vegetables, seaweeds. One of the best ways to supplement calcium is with bonemeal.
How much? Pets who are regularly getting bones may not need additional calcium except in times of specific need such as pregnancy and growth. Give a ¼ teaspoon of bonemeal daily for cats, up to one teaspoon daily for dogs.

Iron is vital for healthy blood, and deficiency can lead to anaemia. Vitamin C increases the uptake of iron in the body.
Good sources? Offal, meat, sardines, egg yolks, dark green leafy vegetables, dried fruit, and the herbs nettle and parsley.
How much? 5mg daily for cats, up to 15mg daily for dogs. Iron is usually included in a multi-mineral complex and can be added separately in times of specific need.

FOOD SUPPLEMENTS

Magnesium is important for healthy bones and teeth, nerve and muscle function. Magnesium is also a great pain-reliever and calmative, along with calcium.
Good sources? Whole grains, dried figs, green leafy vegetables, pulses.
How much? There may not be adequate amounts of magnesium in the diet (due to depleted amounts in the soil), especially in times of specific need. A multi-mineral complex for cats and dogs will usually contain magnesium. Epsom salts are a good source of magnesium; add a pinch daily to a cat's food or two to three pinches for a dog.

Potassium and **sodium** are synergistic and need to be kept in balance. Some pet foods have added salt, which is unnecessary and leads to health problems. The two minerals work together to maintain fluid and electrolyte balance in the cells and tissues. Potassium helps to regulate blood pressure and maintain a normal heartbeat. Ready-made pet foods tend to be low in potassium and high in sodium, and there is rarely a need to supplement sodium in the diet.
Good sources? Dandelions, bananas, avocados, leafy vegetables and garlic are good sources of potassium. Apple cider vinegar adds potassium to the diet and is one of the easiest ways to supplement it.
How much? Add one teaspoon of apple cider vinegar to each pint of water for both cats and dogs.

Zinc is vital for normal growth, the development and health of the reproductive system, the proper functioning of the immune system, healing and healthy skin and coat.
Good sources? Meat, poultry, eggs, shellfish, pumpkin seeds.
How much? 5mg daily for cats, up to 15mg daily for dogs. Zinc is best supplemented as part of a multi-mineral complex and added separately in times of extra need.

Multi-minerals are a convenient way to ensure that your pet is getting the right amount of the above minerals, along with other important trace minerals such as selenium, chromium and manganese. Some of the good-quality ones specifically for dogs and cats include Denes and The Missing Link (and Barley Dog for dogs). During times of specific need you may wish to add specific minerals such as iron for anaemia or zinc in order to fight infection and to heal skin problems.

A combination of bonemeal, alfalfa and kelp will contain all of the above minerals and trace elements and can be added to the diet on a regular basis instead of a multi-mineral complex.

Giving capsules and tablets

If you are using capsules or tablets and you find that your pet won't take them, try opening the capsules up and sprinkling the contents into their food or mixing the contents with a small amount of something they love. Tablets can be crushed and mixed in with food or a tasty treat like butter, fish paste, molasses or sardines.

Liquid supplements can be gently squirted into an animal's mouth using a measuring syringe. Always give your pet an affectionate pat or a treat if they have managed to swallow something they have earlier resisted.

Other valuable supplements

Acidophilus is a form of friendly intestinal bacteria vital for good health. These friendly bacteria are known as probiotics and they inhabit the intestinal system of all animals. The friendly bacteria help pets absorb nutrients, boost the immune system, keep the pH balance of the gut right and eliminate toxins. Always give your pet acidophilus following a course of antibiotics, which tend to wipe out both the unfriendly and the friendly bacteria. Any digestive disturbance like diarrhoea or constipation will benefit from acidophilus. Live yoghurt is also a good source of the friendly bacteria.
How much? One capsule/¼ teaspoon powder daily for cats, two capsules/½ teaspoon powder daily for dogs.

Alfalfa is a rich source of vitamins and minerals, and it also contains over 20 per cent protein. It can be bought in tablet form or powdered and sprinkled over food.

Aloe vera juice is a great detoxifier and bowel cleanser. (Avoid if your pet is pregnant.)

Apple cider vinegar adds potassium (see above) to the diet and is helpful in treating arthritis. It also helps the body to absorb minerals better.
How much? Add one teaspoon per pint of water to your cat or dog's drinking water.

Bonemeal provides calcium to the diet. In the wild, animals eat the bones as well as the flesh of animals, which naturally balances the high phosphorus content of meat with the high calcium content of the bones.
How much? ¼ teaspoon bonemeal daily for cats and up to one teaspoon daily for dogs.

Brewer's yeast is one of the best sources of the whole range of B vitamins and cats and dogs love the taste. It also provides some protein.
How much? ¼–½ teaspoon daily for cats, up to one tablespoon for dogs.

Digestive enzymes enhance the absorption and digestion of food and are useful for older animals, pets with allergies or those in need of digestive support, especially during illness and recovery.
How much? You can use human forms of digestive enzymes in relative amounts.

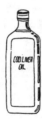

Fish liver oil is a good source of vitamins A and D as well as helping to maintain a healthy heart and circulatory system (see above). Beware of giving your pet too much fish liver oil.
How much? ¼ teaspoon once or twice a week for cats, up to one teaspoon two or three times a week for dogs.

Garlic has a range of health-giving properties, including being an effective anti-viral, anti-bacterial and anti-fungal agent. It fights infections, expels worms and parasites and assists in the healing process.
How much? ¼ clove raw garlic daily for cats, ½–1 clove daily for dogs, mixed in with their meal. Garlic capsules are available if your pet does

not like the taste of raw garlic. Give one capsule every few days for cats, one or two capsules a day for dogs.

Honey is good for the immune system and eases digestive problems. It adds important nutrients to the diet and is a useful addition to a liquid fast. Honey is a natural energiser. It can also be used externally to heal burns.

Kelp is another rich source of vitamins (especially the B vitamins) and minerals (especially potassium) and helps to promote a shiny coat and a healthy skin. It is also a good source of iodine needed by the thyroid to regulate metabolism. It can be bought dried and cooked up or used in powdered form added to food.
How much? ¼ teaspoon daily for cats, up to 1½ teaspoons daily for dogs.

Lecithin granules are a fat emulsifier and help to keep cholesterol and fatty deposits from forming in the body. Lecithin is good for older pets and helps to metabolise fats.
How much? Lecithin granules can be bought in health-food shops and can be sprinkled on food. ¼ teaspoon daily for cats, up to one teaspoon daily for dogs.

Liquid chlorophyll is a great detoxifier as well as providing a rich source of important nutrients to the diet. It is a useful tonic for ill or weak animals and can be added to water or other liquids during a fast.
How much? Chlorophyll is a whole food and will enhance any dietary regime. ½ teaspoon liquid chlorophyll daily for cats, up to three teaspoons daily for dogs.

Psyllium husks are a form of natural vegetable fibre and are brilliant for cleansing the bowel and carrying toxins out of the body. They will help to alleviate a constipated pet.
How much? Psyllium husks come in capsules or as loose powder which can be sprinkled in food. ½ teaspoon daily for cats, up to two teaspoons daily for dogs, as required.

Wheat germ oil is a great source of vitamin E (see above).
How much? One capsule daily for cats, up to four daily for dogs.

Don't panic – you don't have to add these things every day to your pet's food! A good-quality multi-vitamin and mineral complex will supply many of the additional supplements, or use a combination of food sources such as kelp and alfalfa instead. As mentioned, there may be times of specific need when extra nutrients will be required. The above is a guide to how to improve your pet's diet in the way that you and they find most suitable. One of the best all-in-one food supplements for cats and dogs is 'The Missing Link' range which contains a host of valuable nutrients including flax seeds, alfalfa, blackstrap molasses, sunflower seeds, rice bran, dried liver, dried yeast, bonemeal, carrots, fishmeal, kelp, garlic, nettle and spirulina.

Useful information

Where to buy food supplements
Pets shops, pet superstores and health-food shops will have many, if not all, of the supplements listed above.

Other sources
The Nutri Centre
7 Park Crescent
London W1N 3HE
Tel: 0171 436 5122
They also have a mail-order service.

The Missing Link
Savant Distribution Ltd
7 Wayland Croft
Adel
Leeds LS16 8LA
Tel: 0113 230 1993

Many of the herb suppliers will stock alfalfa, kelp, aloe vera and so on. See chapter 11 for details.

CHAPTER FIVE

Acupuncture

钺
久
治
療
狗
和
猫

At-a-glance guide
What is it? Acupuncture involves inserting tiny needles into the animal's body in an effort to stimulate energy flow and bring about self-healing.
What can it help? Most conditions, physical or behavioural, will respond to treatment.
Can you do it yourself? No. Acupuncture should only be done by a qualified veterinary acupuncturist.
Average cost per treatment? In line with standard veterinary fees, depending on the length of the consultation.
Does it hurt? No.

Acupuncture is a form of traditional Chinese medicine which has been used in China for over five thousand years. We know that it has been used on animals for about the same amount of time from the discovery of ancient records and clay models of horses with acupuncture points marked on them.

These days, in China, student vets study acupuncture and Chinese herbs as part of their course.

Acupuncture provides maximum health benefits without the dangerous side effects associated with many modern drugs and surgery

---

What is acupuncture?

Acupuncture is based on the belief that health is determined by having a balanced flow of 'chi' (vital life essence) throughout the body. (In the West we tend to refer to 'chi' as 'life force'.) An imbalance of chi leads to illness, and so by correcting and rebalancing the flow of chi, the body is restored to health. It is a complete system of healing and combines a traditional Chinese diagnosis with treatment using special needles.

The actual treatment involves putting hair-thin needles into specific points along the body in order to stimulate energy flow. These points lie just beneath the surface of the skin and run along energy channels within the body, called meridians. It is by stimulating the energy flow at these specific points that acupuncture aims to treat disease.

The meridians are named after the organs and systems that they have the most effect on, for example, the heart meridian or the kidney meridian. Often a pain at a specific point along a meridian line may indicate that there is a problem with the associated organ, rather than with the place the pain seems to be coming from.

The meridians are not something we can see, in the sense that an anatomist would not tell you there are energy channels in the body. However, the Chinese certainly believe they exist. They believe that the 'Chi' flows along these meridians and gets distributed around the whole body. Chi provides the basic vitality for the body's organs and tissues and promotes good health by maintaining body harmony.

What disease, or the result of the disease process, does is to interfere with the flow of Chi. Acupuncture can influence the energy flow and normalise it, returning the body to a healthy, balanced state where it can ultimately heal itself.

'The principles of acupuncture don't sit easily on conventional Western shoulders because you have the idea of "life forces" and "lines of energy" which run through the body. Funnily enough, Western medicine has found that an awful lot of these energy lines are allied to nerve pathways.'
Alasdair MacFarlane Govan, BVMS, MRCVS

Do animals enjoy acupuncture?

Acupuncture does not hurt and most vets report that dogs and cats do not seem to mind it and often fall asleep during their treatment. The ones that do not like it are usually animals that do not like being handled anyway. Remember, animals do not have the same psychological fear of needles as some humans do!

Using acupuncture on animals

Acupuncture works in exactly the same way with animals as it does with people except that the method of diagnosis is slightly different. An acupuncturist working with people will often ask detailed questions as part of their diagnosis – which you obviously cannot do with pets! However, to use acupuncture fully with animals you still have to make what is called a 'traditional Chinese diagnosis'.

Making a diagnosis

This involves looking at various different aspects of the animal. This could be looking at the coating on the tongue, feeling the animal's pulse, looking at its general condition and observing its behaviour. They may also ask you about your pet's sleeping and eating habits, digestion and urine and so on.

Many vets will also look to see whether it is more what is called a 'yang' animal or a 'yin' animal. The yang animal is an extrovert, bouncy type of animal, whereas a yin animal is more of a quiet type. The Chinese believe that good health depends on the proper balance between yin and yang – two opposing forces, or opposite poles of energy – and an imbalance can result in ill health.

During the diagnosis they will be looking at all of these characteristics to work out what the 'normal' energy of the body is. Taking the pulse gives an idea of the yin-yang element as well as giving an idea of the 'character' of the energy and the strength of the flow. They will also ask you what your pet is normally like, because animals do change a bit when they walk into the surgery. Generally, with veterinary acupuncture, you can expect quite a lot of owner participation, more so perhaps than with orthodox veterinary treatment.

Some vets will not have the time to use acupuncture in a truly holistic way and use what is called recipe acupuncture. This is where certain points are known to be good for certain symptoms and conditions and it does not rely on first making a traditional Chinese diagnosis. However, to use acupuncture to its full healing capacity you really have to make a complete Chinese diagnosis and follow the principles of holistic treatment, treating the whole being rather than just the disease symptoms.

Most veterinary acupuncturists will probably also look over the animal with their orthodox hat on because there are benefits from both Western and Chinese diagnoses, and in some cases it may be best to combine modern drugs with acupuncture.

Acupuncture points in dogs and cats

There are hundreds and hundreds of acupuncture points all over dogs and cats but only about 30 points are commonly used, and not all of these would be used in the same session. More usually, a vet works on five or fewer points at a time.

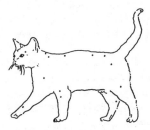

Acupuncure needles are inserted at specific points in order to balance the flow of energy

Animals can be treated either standing up or lying down, depending on the vet's preference and which points are being used. Often animals feel quite sleepy during their treatment. The needles may be left in for up to half an hour, but as with all complementary treatments there are no hard and fast rules about how long a session might take. It depends on the animal and what is happening with the energy. Every animal will respond differently.

Why choose acupuncture for my pet?

For a start, you are not giving your pet anything that is going to give it nasty side effects like some drugs can – especially if your pet is going to be on the drugs long term. For example, chronic, painful arthritis can mean that they are on steroid drugs for a number of years. In the end these can be harmful to one thing or another, usually the liver and kidneys. Acupuncture does not have adverse side effects and treats the body as a whole. Many animals also get a feeling of well-being from the acupuncture which they do not necessarily get from drugs. Acupuncture is an holistic treatment in the sense that although you might have taken your animal in with a particular problem, there might be other underlying things which will also benefit from the acupuncture. This is the advantage of using acupuncture as a complete treatment, rather than the 'recipe acupuncture' of symptom relief.

Animals can also benefit greatly from acupuncture when they are ready to die. It has been found that death is often more peaceful and occurs with less suffering if the animal has acupuncture treatment.

What can be treated with acupuncture?

Acupuncture is very effective in certain cases and less so in others. Often the cases in which it is not so effective are ones where it is used as a last-ditch attempt to cure something.

'Unfortunately a lot of people try all aspects of Western medicine first, and then they say, "Nothing is working. I've heard you can use acupuncture in animals, so let's give it a go." By the time the animal begins treatment it may already be too late to stimulate its own natural healing powers.'
Alasdair MacFarlane Govan, BVMS, MRCVS

Acupuncture is as much a preventative medicine as it is a potential cure, and the sooner an animal is brought for treatment the more likely it is to make a full recovery. With acupuncture the emphasis has always been on prevention.

The emphasis of traditional Chinese medicine is more on prevention than cure and works on the principle that it's better to shut the stable door before the horse has bolted.

Vets who use acupuncture find that the kinds of conditions it can best help include:

- Chronic conditions like arthritis, rheumatism, back problems, gastrointestinal diseases

- Musculo-skeletal problems such as hip dysplasia, slipped disc, problems with joints, spinal problems, locomotive problems, some types of paralysis and injuries

- Pain relief generally and after surgery. Acupuncture has been found to be effective when morphine has not. It stimulates the body's own natural pain-killing chemicals.

- Respiratory problems

- Skin conditions, allergic dermatitis, hair loss and other types of skin problems

- Neurological problems such as epilepsy, anxiety and behavioural problems

- Urinary control and kidney disorders

- Reproductive disorders. Vets have reported success with treating the heat cycle of bitches, bitches who are continuously having false pregnancies or very short heat cycles, and balancing hormones.

- Liver problems

'We often use it for liver problems, because there is not much else you can do anyway. It really does tend to work very well, because there is a very strong energy path from an area of the spine down to the liver.'
Helen Gould, BVetMed, MRCVS

- Appetite problems. It is great for encouraging eating, especially with cats, as they can tend to go off their food after surgery.

- Hormonal problems. Almost all the endocrine glands, such as the reproductive organs and the thyroid, can be

THE NATURAL WAY FOR DOGS AND CATS

influenced. Blood sugar control can be normalised in diabetic animals.

For specific ailments, see chapter 16.

Case histories

'I treated a basset hound who when he first came for acupuncture was walking on his hocks. He had dreadful back legs and his owners had given up on him. He had very slack joints and poor muscular tone and I treated him for about three to four weeks. The dog is actually walking quite well now. It has been to shows and even been placed. That's a success, without a doubt.'

'Another lady brought two dogs here and they both had spondylosis of the spine. They were slowly but surely losing the power of all their limbs and were heading to be put down. They were sisters and had been referred to me by another vet. The vet the owner went to had been taking serial X-rays and could see the spondylosis getting worse and worse. She brought the dogs for acupuncture about once or twice a week for six months and from the time of starting the acupuncture the spondylosis just slowly started to disappear. Those two dogs got better and never needed any more treatment, and that was it.'

Alasdair MacFarlane Govan, BVMS, MRCVS

How many treatments will my pet need?

It really depends on the individual cat or dog. If you are dealing with a chronic case (a long-term problem) it can take quite a number of treatments before you see any effect. It is important to remember that natural healing methods often take longer to work than drug treatments. Some vets may put a limit on the amount of treatment they will give if there has been no improvement, because it may be that the chance of recovery is slight or that it will take too long. Having said that, most cats and dogs will respond after just one or two treatments.

With acute (short-term) conditions there may be a fairly dramatic response because the energy has not been out of balance for as long and can therefore be corrected more quickly than in chronic situations. With a long-term chronic condition like arthritis, the acupuncture is not really treating the arthritis. What it is doing is relieving the pain and letting the animal feel better about everything.

This is one of the benefits of acupuncture – it improves quality of life in a situation where the disease process cannot actually be reversed, and it also helps to slow down the disease process. In cases like this you might have to take your pet for a booster dose whenever it needs it, which will vary depending on the animal and the speed of degeneration. Some animals may go a month between appointments, some may go two months, and it is not unusual for them to go as long as six months.

Home use?

Acupuncture does not lend itself to being carried out in the home and has to be practised by a qualified vet. There are far too many risks involved in untrained hands, and it is not a therapy that can be done at home in the same way that the flower essences and homoeopathy can. However, more and more vets these days are training in animal acupuncture; it should therefore be possible to find one in your local area (see 'Where to find a veterinary acupuncturist' at the end of this chapter).

Can acupuncture be used with other therapies?

Like many other forms of complementary medicine, acupuncture is a complete system that stands on its own and should be respected as such. It is best not to use lots of different therapies and treatments at once. Combining healing with acupuncture, for example, would not be a good idea, since they are both working with subtle energy and can interfere with each other, but a more physical treatment, like herbal medicine, would be all right to use at the same time. Acupuncture also complements conventional medicine very well and can be used to enhance its effects.

'I think really the best use for veterinary acupuncture is to integrate it more with Western medicine, and I feel that more vets should use it. For instance, you can inject vitamins at acupuncture points and get an enhanced effect. You can inject antibiotics at a point that will give pain relief and stimulate healing. So you can inject your antibiotic normally and put a little bit of it at the acupuncture sites to get a better effect.'
Helen Gould, BVetMed, MRCVS

The future of veterinary acupuncture

There is a growing interest in veterinary acupuncture from pet owners who prefer to use natural treatments and remedies on their pets. Many vets too feel that they cannot always adequately treat some conditions with orthodox Western medicine and have added acupuncture to their practice to help them with those conditions.

This growing understanding and respect for acupuncture and its place in veterinary medicine has led to it being increasingly integrated into standard veterinary medicine.

Laser acupuncture

This is another way of stimulating the acupuncture points in people and animals. It involves using a low-intensity laser and it is often used to heal wounds and reduce swelling.

Electro acupuncture

This involves attaching electrodes to the acupuncture needles so that small electric currents can be passed through the needles into the acupuncture points.

Acupressure

This is the pressing of the acupuncture point with a finger or thumb. Sometimes it is useful when an animal needs treatment several times a day; obviously a vet cannot see them that often, so they might explain to the owner where the point is and get them to press when necessary. This works well for animals who are in a lot of pain or go into spasms of pain, because the owner can do something to help immediately. Acupressure should only be done under veterinary guidance and is not something that people should do off their own bat, since it can cause other problems or make the pain worse if the wrong points are used.

Useful information

Where to find a veterinary acupuncturist
   The Association of British Veterinary Acupuncture
   Handcross
   Haywards Heath
   West Sussex RH17 6BD
   Tel: 01444 400213

Contact Jill Hewson for a list of qualified veterinary acupuncturists in the UK.

Further reading

Four Paws, Five Directions by Cheryl Schwartz, DVM; Celestial Arts Publishing
Canine Acupressure by Nancy Zidonis and Marie Soderburg

CHAPTER SIX

Aromatherapy

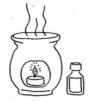

At-a-glance guide

What is it? The use of plant essential oils to treat disease.

What can it help? All sorts of problems, physical, mental and emotional. Also good for first-aid use.

Can you do it yourself? Yes. Essential oils are easy to use and are widely available.

Is it safe? Yes, when used correctly and in the appropriate quantities.

Average cost of treatment? The cost of individual oils varies; some are relatively inexpensive, others are quite expensive. Treatment from a professional aromatherapist will be in keeping with standard consultation fees.

Aromatherapy for animals is the art and science of using plant essential oils to treat both the emotional body and the physical body of animals. It takes into consideration the whole animal, so you are not just treating one specific symptom of illness. The oils work to support the animal's whole being in an effort to rid it of disease.

Like other holistic treatments, aromatherapy puts great emphasis on prevention being better than cure. Essential oils have a positive effect on an animal's whole being – mind, body and spirit – and leave no toxic residue in the way that synthetic drugs do.

What are essential oils?

Essential oils are aromatic essences extracted from a wide variety of trees and plants, such as eucalyptus, pine, geranium, lavender and jasmine. The essential oils are contained in tiny glands in the plants and have potent therapeutic properties. They could even be described as the very 'spirit' or 'soul' of a plant.

How do they work?

Exactly how essential oils work is something of a mystery, but we know they have active medicinal properties. They seem to work energetically, like the flower essences, and can positively influence an animal's vital force. The energy of the oils interacts with the energy of the animal to produce a healing effect. When an animal's vital force becomes weakened or impaired in some way, disease often follows. You get outward signs that something is wrong, such as a heart condition or a behavioural problem. Yet the root cause of the illness may be physical, emotional or mental, and by rebalancing the vital force, the body is brought back into harmony and health. When you treat an animal with an essential oil, the healing properties are drawn to whichever part of the body is out of balance and in need of healing. By increasing the animal's vital force, its own powers of self-healing are stimulated. Essential oils have a fast-acting therapeutic action on the body and some, like lavender and lemon, are adaptogenic, which means they are able to adapt to what the body needs at the time.

Essential oils work to support every aspect of an animal.

Healing properties of essential oils

Not all oils have the same properties, but in general essential oils are antiseptic and detoxifying, and they help to strengthen the immune system and regulate metabolism. They all contain active chemical constituents, and in many cases modern medicine has taken the individual chemical constituents from the oils and made them into a patented product. For example, thymol, which is used for treating throat and mouth conditions, is extracted from thyme. Thymol is a patented product using one small part of the oil.

'In taking a small part of that oil away and making it into a product in its own right, you lose a lot of the synergistic process of that oil, which is all the parts working together to form the cure. So, to go back to the concept of holism, looking at the whole animal, I think

you need to use the whole product to get an effective cure.'
Sarah Fisher, aromatherapist

Essential oils have powerful antiseptic, anti-viral, anti-bacterial and anti-fungal properties. They are detoxifying and revitalising, anti-inflammatory, pain-relieving, relaxing, soothing and anti-depressant. They can regulate the nervous system and the hormonal system and have a diuretic effect on the body. They can also be used to heal injuries and repel insects.

Because of these wide-ranging curative properties, essential oils can be used to treat a variety of conditions and are especially effective in boosting the immune system, increasing resistance to disease and fighting infection.

Plant essential oils are usually extracted by a process of distillation to capture the healing essence. Plant essential oils are very concentrated, which makes them extremely potent even in tiny amounts.

Using aromatherapy with animals
Aromatherapy could be described as a 'branch' of herbal medicine, but, unlike herbs, it is only in the past few decades that aromatherapy has been used on animals – and only very recently has it become a popular treatment, particularly for dogs, cats and horses.

Most animals love aromatherapy, but if this is not the case, the treatment should not be used.

How to use essential oils
Essential oils can be used in a variety of ways, the most common being massage and inhalation.

Baths This is a useful way of using essential oils to combat fleas and other external parasites, and to soothe and heal skin problems. Add a few drops of your chosen oil to water and bathe your pet.

Compresses A compress of essential oils and water helps to relieve bruising, muscle pain and skin problems. Add one or two drops of essential oil to a bowl of warm water. Soak a piece of cotton in the water, put it over the area to be treated and leave the compress in place for up to an hour at a time.

Inhalation Essential oils can be absorbed by inhalation using burners, diffusers or vaporisers which make the essential oils airborne. This is the best way to treat cats, since they are often sensitive to having oils massaged into their skin. Treatment by inhalation is ideal for all kinds of respiratory problems and is great for disinfecting places where several animals are kept in a small area, such as kennels and catteries. With infections, like kennel cough and feline flu, using oils in a diffuser is very appropriate, because you minimise the spread of that disease to other animals.

A diffuser has an electrical motor which pumps a fine spray of essential oils into the air. The oils can be used undiluted. Diffusers do not heat the oils, which makes this method the most attractive. Burners heat the essential oils by a candle, or you can use a burner ring placed on top of a warm light bulb. When using burners, dilute the essential oil with water. A vaporiser has an electrical heater and the oils can be used undiluted.

Treatment by inhalation should be done twice a day for a week.

Massage Diluted oils can be gently massaged into an animal's skin, where they are very quickly absorbed. Most pets enjoy being touched and find massage relaxing and soothing. Massage is also toning and harmonising and is a good form of treatment for pets who need to be calmed. Touch is very therapeutic and most pets love it. Add one or two drops of your chosen oil to a teaspoon of almond oil or vegetable oil and lightly massage into the skin for around five minutes. For most complaints and conditions you can do this twice a day for a week.

Be careful about using aromatherapy on the skin of cats because they can be hypersensitive (this is why a lot of cats have problems with flea collars and flea powders). When you are working with cats, it is best to use the essential oils in a burner, diffuser or vaporiser so that the cat is inhaling the aroma and getting the healing benefits that way.

Neat Lavender and tea tree oils can sometimes be used neat (undiluted) on burns, cuts, grazes, bites and stings. However, this can cause irritation, so it is best to dilute the essential oils just a little in almond oil or vegetable oil.

Taken internally Internal use of aromatherapy is fairly controversial and is practised much more in France than it is in the UK. Do not give your pet oils to eat unless you are experienced in using essential oils and know exactly what effect you are hoping to achieve. Any internal use of essential oils should be under the guidance of your vet or an experienced aromatherapist. This is because essential oils are very concentrated and it is easy to give an overdose and actually harm your pet. Having said that, taking essential oils internally can be most beneficial for digestive problems, internal parasites and other things. You can mix the essential oils with wheatgerm oil, which is high in vitamin E, and just add it to their food – but always be mindful of the potency of essential oils.

Dosage
Essential oils are very potent and should always be diluted when used directly on the skin or taken internally. Add two or three drops of essential oil to two teaspoons of a base oil such as almond oil or vegetable oil. You can mix different essential oils and use up to three in the same blend.

What can aromatherapy help?

- Digestive problems, allergies

- Emotional problems, nervousness, stress, anxiety

- Skin complaints, parasites

- Respiratory problems

- Car sickness

- Arthritis, rheumatism, sprains and strains

- Viral complaints such as kennel cough and feline flu

- Infections

For specific ailments, see chapter 16.

First-aid use (also see chapter 15)

Aromatherapy is great for first-aid use. For example, you can use tea tree and lavender or any of the antiseptic oils in a dilution for cuts, grazes and burns. In cases of shock, lavender is a really good carminative. You can massage lavender into your pet's ears – there is a 'shock point' at the tip of the ear which means you can combine the effect of the essential oil with the calming effect of massaging the ears.

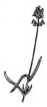

Using essential oils yourself

Although each animal is an individual and should be treated holistically, some oils are known to work well for particular conditions (see chapters 15 and 16).

Is it safe?

Aromatherapy oils are very concentrated and need to be used with care. They are safe if you are aware of the properties of the oils and use them in the correct dilutions. They are nearly always used in a diluted form to prevent overdosing and irritation. Some of the essential oils are harmful during pregnancy; ones to avoid include basil, rosemary, thyme, sage, clary sage and juniper.

The fact that they are natural does not make them safe. You can overdose with essential oils and the reactions can be severe. For example, if you are using rosemary on a dog that has suffered from epilepsy, it can provoke an epileptic fit. Some of the citrus oils that are used to keep bugs away are photo-sensitising for animals and can cause sunburn and irritation.

Always keep the oils away from an animal's eyes. If you have an allergic pet, first do a patch test on a healthy part of their body using a diluted oil and wait for at least half an hour to see if there is any adverse reaction.

Always follow professional advice unless you have a good

understanding of the individual oils and what they can do – because, without meaning to, you could overdose the animal and potentially cause more problems than you are trying to cure.

'I do think there is definitely a place for using aromatherapy on animals, but it needs to be reasonably well researched and pet owners need to know what they are doing before they just run to the chemist to get the oils and administer them to their pet.'
Sarah Fisher, aromatherapist

Consulting an aromatherapist

For more complicated or serious cases, always seek the advice of your vet or ask them to refer you to a qualified aromatherapist. If your vet is not open to holistic treatment, find one who is. Usually a homoeopathic vet will be a lot more supportive of other methods of natural healing. Most qualified aromatherapists belong to a governing body; you can therefore contact one of these and ask for a list of members who work with animals in your area (see 'Useful information' for contact addresses and telephone numbers).

During a consultation the practitioner will take a full case history of your pet and ask about sleeping and eating habits to get a complete picture of the disease process in the animal. They may also ask you to continue the treatment at home between appointments, using a diffuser or by giving your pet a massage with the appropriate essential oils.

Cost of treatment

Treatment from an aromatherapist is usually in keeping with homoeopathic vets and other natural therapists.

Response to treatment

The effects can be immediate and long-lasting, but asking how long the treatment takes is a bit like asking 'how long is a piece of string?'. Every animal is different and much depends on its age, general health and how long the condition has been around. A few days may effect a cure, and a period of three to six weeks is usually long enough to restore balance to the animal's system. Remember that a healthy lifestyle and a natural preservative-free diet will enhance the healing potential of aromatherapy.

Case histories

'I treated a dog that had a lot of emotional issues, and I used frankincense with a little bit of lavender for a massage rub into her tummy. She had a lot of fear problems, like a fear of letting go of old patterns of behaviour. She liked the smell of the two oils; frankincense and lavender were the oils that she was most drawn to. It is sometimes a case of watching the animal and letting them pick what they want. Frankincense is really good for dogs who have had abuse problems, because it helps them to let go of the past.'

'A cat that I treated had feline leukaemia and had been damaged as a result. Using very weak dilutions, I used one drop of frankincense and one drop of jasmine to 10mls of vegetable oil and rubbed that on his chest. I asked the owner to continue the treatment at home and to be really careful about not rubbing it right into the skin. I applied it once and said that she should see how it goes over three days. The owner phoned to say she had done it once more and he never sneezed again. Other cats with feline flu could take longer – it depends on how long the illness has been there and what other weaknesses there are – but normally you would get to see an improvement within a couple of days.'
Sarah Fisher, aromatherapist

Is aromatherapy compatible with other treatments?

It is compatible with most other natural therapies and orthodox treatment. It could work against homoeopathy, though, and most homoeopaths and aromatherapists will agree between them not to use the two together, because they can cancel each other out. It is probably best not to mix aromatherapy and homoeopathy, but instead to allow each treatment to have its maximum benefit.

Aromatherapy medicine chest for cats and dogs

Eucalyptus Eucalyptus is antiseptic, anti-viral and decongestant. It is a good essential oil if you are dealing with bacterial or viral infections and it can be used in a burner or diffuser in the animal's room or in a cattery or kennel. Eucalyptus eases respiratory difficulties. Used with massage it helps ease rheumatism and arthritis. Eucalyptus essential oil is extracted from the leaves and mature branches of the eucalyptus tree.
Cost: Inexpensive.

Geranium Geranium is soothing, refreshing and relaxing. Geranium soothes skin irritations and helps to heal burns and minor abrasions. The essential oil is extracted from the whole plant, before it flowers.
Cost: Inexpensive.

Lavender Lavender is one of the most useful essential oils and is a must for any first-aid kit. It is good for bacterial and viral problems, it is soothing and helps to heal sore, inflamed areas. Lavender acts as a flea deterrent, and soothes burns. It is calming and sedative. It is extracted from lavender pods.
Cost: Inexpensive.

Marjoram Marjoram is very good at killing airborne bacteria and has strong antibiotic properties. It helps to combat anxiety and stress. It can be used in massage to treat strained muscles and aching limbs. The essential oil is extracted from the flowering tops and leaves of the herb.
Cost: Fairly expensive.

Melissa Melissa is very good for when a pet has died or has had to be put down. Burning melissa oil at these times can help the other animals in the household to come to terms with the death. Melissa is also good for treating nervous conditions and stress.
Cost: Expensive.

Peppermint Peppermint oil is a good digestive tonic and has anti-spasmodic properties, making it useful for colic and other digestive complaints. You can use it on an animal's bedding to keep fleas away. Spray the bed with a solution of peppermint oil, vodka (to dilute the essential oil) and water. Do not put undiluted peppermint oil straight on to their bed because it will go rancid. Peppermint is very cooling and refreshing, which makes it particularly appealing during the summer. The oil comes from the leaves of the plant.
Cost: Inexpensive.

Tea tree Tea tree is another of the most useful oils and, like lavender, it is a must for any first-aid kit. It boosts the immune system and is well known for its antiseptic, anti-bacterial, anti-fungal and anti-viral properties. Tea tree is also very good for using as a wash. If you have had a sick animal, you can cleanse the area with tea tree so that other animals do not get the sickness as well. It is good for dandruff and skin disorders including burns, insect bites and warts. The essential oil is distilled from the leaves and twigs of this common Australian tree. Cost: Inexpensive.

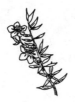

Buying the oils

Many essential oils on the market are not 'pure' essential oils but are blended. Even those that claim to be 'pure essential oil' are likely to be pure oils that have been mixed with another cheaper oil. For example, a good rose oil should cost over two hundred pounds for about 1–2 mls! However, most of the commonly used essential oils are inexpensive, and if you do not use pure oils you cannot expect to get a curative result. Synthetic copies simply do not work. Always buy essential oils from reputable sources who specialise in aromatherapy oils for practitioners (see suppliers at the end of the chapter).

Storing the oils

Stored correctly, essential oils should last for a few years. Because they are sensitive to heat, light, plastic and air, they need to be stored with care. Essential oils should be stored in tinted glass bottles and kept away from heat and strong sunlight.

Useful information

Further reading
Veterinary Aromatherapy by Nelly Grosjean; The C.W. Daniel Company Limited

Where to find an aromatherapist to treat your pet
International Federation of Aromatherapists
Stamford House
2–4 Chiswick High Road
London W4 1TH
Tel: 0181 742 2606

ISPA
(International Society of Professional Aromatherapists)
82 Ashby Road
Hinckley
Leicestershire LE10 1SN
Tel: 01455 637987

Suppliers of essential oils and aromatherapy products for animals

New Seasons
The Old Post Office
Lockinge
Oxon OX12 8PA
Tel: 01235 821110

New Seasons stock a range of ready-made aromatherapy products for dogs and cats, such as ear drops, bedding spray, skin creams and shampoos.

Essentially Oils Ltd.
8–10 Mount Farm
Junction Road
Churchill
Chipping Norton
Oxon OX7 6NP
Tel: 01608 659544

Suppliers of pure essential oils, base oils, burners, vaporisers, diffusers, books and so on.

CHAPTER SEVEN

Biochemical Tissue Salts

At-a-glance guide
What are they? Tiny sugar milk tablets containing potentised mineral salts.
What can they help? Many minor physical and behavioural problems.
Can you do it yourself? Yes. They are perfectly safe and there is no danger of overdosing.
Cost? The tissue salts are relatively inexpensive.

Biochemical tissue salts are potentised preparations of 12 of the most common mineral salts found in the body. They were first developed by a Dr Wilhelm Schuessler, who believed that many diseases were caused by a lack of one or more of these 12 vital mineral salts. For example, a lack of calcium phosphate would lead to teeth problems, and a deficiency of magnesium phosphate would affect the nerves and muscles.

The use of tissue salts is really a branch of homoeopathy. While homoeopathy cures 'like with like', tissue salts treat disease by correcting mineral imbalances inside the body's cells which helps to restore health. Tissue salts are made only from mineral sources, whereas homoeopathic remedies are made from animal, mineral and vegetable sources. (It may be helpful to read chapter 12 as well, which gives a fuller understanding of how homoeopathy works and the thinking behind it.)

Using tissue salts with animals
Tissue salts have been used successfully on animals for over 100 years. Animals often respond very quickly and there is no danger of overdosing or of nasty side effects.

63

Animals have always been instinctive about their health and will naturally try to restore imbalances and deficiencies of important nutrients. This is why they sometimes have peculiar appetites for surprising foods. Research shows that some ailments in animals are directly linked to mineral and trace-element deficiencies.

How do tissue salts work?

The potentised mineral salt takes on healing properties over and above that of the material substance from which it was made. It is like a supercharged version of the original substance – this is in essence the principle of how tissue salts work. They restore the healthy functioning of the cells by stimulating the body's own powers of recovery.

What can they help?

- Digestive problems

- First-aid cases such as burns and wounds

- Behavioural problems, anxiety

- Skin and coat problems

- Chronic conditions like rheumatism and arthritis

For specific ailments, see chapter 16.
For first-aid use, see chapter 15.

Treating your pet yourself at home

The key to successful treatment is to match the symptoms to the remedy. Unlike homoeopathy, which builds a whole picture of the disease, the tissue salts are based on the theory that a specific symptom indicates that a specific tissue salt is needed.

Tissue salts are easy to use and there are only 12 basic remedies to choose from.

Giving tissue salts to your pet

The remedies need to be given away from meal times and can be put straight into your cat or dog's mouth. Because they are soft, they dissolve almost immediately so there is little chance of your pet spitting them out again!

Tissue salts can also be used externally for cuts and wounds. For example, iron phosphate tablets can be crushed and rubbed into the affected part (after it has been cleaned). Alternatively, you can dissolve the tablets in sterilised water and make a paste to rub straight on to the skin.

The 12 mineral salts

Calcium fluoride (calc. fluor.) Maintains the elasticity of tissues, improves the strength of the heart muscle. Good for arthritis. Strengthens teeth.

Calcium phosphate (calc. phos.) Constituent of bones and teeth. Helpful in cases of bone healing, indigestion, itching skin.

Calcium sulphate (calc. sulph.) Blood constituent. Good for skin problems, suppurating burns and wounds.

Iron phosphate (ferr. phos.) Minor respiratory disorders, blood stream oxygenation. Good in cases of inflammation, rheumatism, first stages of fever, wounds, sprains and strains.

Potassium chloride (kali. mur.) Minor respiratory disorders. Cold symptoms, second stages of inflammation, rheumatism and swelling, warts, burns, cystitis, constipation.

Potassium phosphate (kali. phos.) Soothes the nerves. Useful for irritability, anxiety, stress, cystitis, itching skin, bad breath, travel sickness.

Potassium sulphate (kali. sulph.) Maintains a healthy skin and coat. Good for hair loss, eczema and dandruff.

Magnesium phosphate (mag. phos.) Soft-tissue salt. Good for cramp, colic, cystitis, flatulence. A nerve tonic.

Sodium chloride (nat. mur.) Important for fluid balance. Helpful in cases of watery discharges, e.g. diarrhoea, runny nose. Also good for dandruff, eczema and infertility. Can be applied topically to bites and stings.

Sodium phosphate (nat. phos.) Acid neutraliser. Good for digestive problems.

Sodium sulphate (nat. sulph.) Balances fluids in the body. Used for queasiness, digestive upsets, vomiting, rheumatism.

Silicon dioxide (silica) Skin and coat conditioner. Good for hair loss. General cleanser.

You can also get combination remedies of two or more tissue salts. For example, combination M for nervousness, anxiety and stress contains calc. phos., kali phos. and ferr. phos.

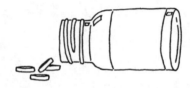

Dosage

Like homoeopathic remedies, the tissue salts are tiny sugar milk tablets which contain the potentised mineral salt. The dosage is the same for dogs and cats and there is no danger of overdosing. Any excess will be eliminated by the body and, since they are harmless, if you prescribe the wrong remedy it will not have any adverse effects. However, like all natural remedies, it is always best to use them in the recommended dose:

ACUTE, short-term problems: two to four tablets three times a day. In severe cases, two to four tablets can be given every half-hour until the symptoms lessen.

CHRONIC, long-term conditions may need to be treated for a number of weeks. Give two tablets, twice a day.

Always consult your vet if your pet's condition is serious.

How quickly do they work?

With acute, short-term conditions your pet may improve within a matter of hours, especially if the tablets are being given every half an hour or so. It can take much longer to notice improvements in long-term conditions, and it can be as long as six months in some cases. A lot depends on the animal's age and breed, but in general the longer a condition has been around, the longer it will take to heal. Do not expect an instant cure; mineral salts, like other natural forms of treatment, work by gradually and gently restoring the body to health and harmony.

Storage

The tablets will keep for about three years if stored in a cool, dry place away from strong light.

Can they be used with other treatments and remedies?

The biochemical tissue salts complement other treatments and therapies well.

Useful information

Where to buy biochemical tissue salts

These are widely available from health-food shops and chemists and are made by New Era.

Further reading

A Guide to Biochemical Tissue Salts by Dr Andrew Stanway; Van Dyke Books

CHAPTER EIGHT

McTimoney Chiropractic

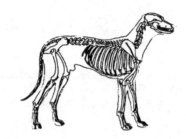

At-a-glance guide
What is it? Gentle manipulation of the spine and skeletal system using only the hands.
What can it help? All kinds of musculo-skeletal problems.
Average cost per treatment? Variable, but usually in keeping with standard veterinary fees.
Can you do it yourself? No. Treatment by professionally trained chiropractors only (see 'Where to find a McTimoney chiropractor').
Is it safe? Yes, in trained hands.

McTimoney chiropractic is a hands-on treatment which aligns and balances an animal's musculo-skeletal system. Much of the treatment concentrates on the spine and its effect on the animal's central nervous system. Just like us, dogs and cats get back, neck, pelvic and musculo-skeletal problems, and so they too can be helped by chiropractic.

Like osteopathy, chiropractic probably has its roots in the hands of the old bonesetters, until it became an established form of treatment in the 1890s. McTimoney chiropractic is a branch of the original chiropractic methods and was developed by a man called John McTimoney. It was he who first adapted chiropractic techniques to suit animals, which is why most practitioners treating animals today are trained in McTimoney chiropractic. That was in the 1950s, and since then many McTimoney chiropractors have turned their attention to treating animals.

Practitioners use only their hands to treat, and the McTimoney method is known for its gentleness and simplicity, which means that animals accept it quite readily. It is a natural, non-invasive treatment and is quite safe in experienced hands. McTimoney chiropractic takes account of the animal's whole body and the deeper effects that structural problems can have on internal organs and systems.

How does it work?

McTimoney chiropractic aims to align and balance the animal's musculo-skeletal system using light and gentle manipulation techniques. The musculo-skeletal system refers to the whole of the body's structure – the bones, joints, muscles, ligaments and tendons.

The chiropractor uses gentle manipulations which cause the animal's own muscles and ligaments to bring the bones back into place. By adjusting any misalignments using swift but gentle thrusts, the animal's muscles respond and pull the vertebrae back into the correct position naturally.

In chiropractic, the spine is a particularly important area of treatment and plays much more than just a structural and supportive role. It also houses and protects the central nervous system. The animal's nerve supply goes right the way down the spine, and if a nerve gets pinched or trapped, the electrical impulse cannot be carried down the nerve pathways properly. Therefore a major organ, like the heart or the liver, can be adversely affected. Treatment can remove tension and relieve pain. Chiropractic treats the deeper cause of symptoms and is therefore a whole-body treatment.

'If you think of the nerve supply as being rather like a hosepipe, depending on the amount of pressure you put on it, you can either speed up the water or slow it down. The nerve supply is exactly the same: a little bit of pressure can speed up the nerve supply and lead to overactivity of that particular organ, or it can cause underactivity if it's pressed a bit harder.'
The Hon. Richard Arthur, McTimoney chiropractor

If anything damages the spine, or if vertebrae get out of alignment, it can affect the rest of the body too. If there is pressure on the nerves, they cannot carry out their proper function – and this can lead to disharmony and disease. Because of this, when chiropractors work on an animal's body, seemingly unrelated internal symptoms may be cured as a result of the spinal manipulation.

'I won't go ahead and treat an animal for, say, a kidney problem, but I may well relieve it incidentally while I am treating the spine.'
The Hon. Richard Arthur, McTimoney chiropractor

Realigning and rebalancing the animal's body not only restores mobility but also takes any undue pressure off the nerve pathways which are connected to all its major organs and systems.

McTimoney chiropractors believe that most disorders originate from a lack of nerve supply, and chiropractic enables the cause of this lack of supply to be addressed by correcting any misalignments.

Making a diagnosis
Usually an animal will already have seen a vet to get the initial diagnosis before being referred to a chiropractor. The chiropractor will then take account of the vet's diagnosis and discuss this with you, as well as asking you various questions about your pet. Then he or she will make a physical check of the animal, both by looking at it and by feeling it with his hands.

The animal is thoroughly checked in this way for possible misalignments, with particular regard to the spine and the pelvis. The chiropractor will check the vertebrae to see what alignment or misalignment there is. Relevant joints and muscles (which may be in spasm) are also checked, as is the animal's range of movements.

Treating animals
Once the source of the problem has been discovered, the area is treated with gentle but swift manipulations to correct any misalignment and reduce muscle spasm. The practitioner will use only his hands in a gentle and non-intrusive way. McTimoney chiropractic is famed for its light touch that almost teases the joints and muscles to respond, rather than forcing them to do so. This ensures that animals do not suffer any discomfort during treatment.

What can be treated?

- Lameness

- Uncharacteristic changes in mobility

- Limb-dragging or irregular limb action

- Paralysis

- Joints out of place following a fall or accident

- Stiffness

- Trapped nerves, pain

- Spinal problems

- General musculo-skeletal problems

Symptoms of musculo-skeletal problems

- Crying out when getting up

- Difficulty climbing stairs or climbing in or out of a car

- Reluctance to exercise

- Shying away from being stroked along the back

- Movement unusual for that particular animal

- Favouring the use of one limb over another

- Swelling, stiffness, lameness

- Irritability

Dogs

Many breeds of dog are worked hard, especially greyhounds, and this high performance and high expectation can take its toll. Animals like these may often need regular chiropractic treatment, as competitive racing places a lot of extra strain on their musculo-skeletal system. Common causes of problems in greyhounds are negotiating tight corners and continually running in one direction.

Other breeds, like dachshunds and basset hounds and those with long backs, can be prone to spinal problems. Simply going up and down an awkward staircase or being overweight can put too much extra pressure on a potentially weak area.

Cats

Cats are not asked to perform in the way that many dogs are, but they are just as likely to suffer from musculo-skeletal problems if they have been in a road accident or have fallen from a height.

For specific ailments, see chapter 16.

Preventative treatment

Any animal asked to perform beyond the normal life of a pet – like greyhounds, police dogs and sporting dogs – can benefit from preventative treatment. Regular fine-tuning of animals' structure helps them to perform at their best. The joints and muscles of hard-working animals can also wear out more quickly; regular treatment is therefore a good way of taking care of your animal.

How many treatments?

It is hard to be precise, since the effectiveness of the treatment depends on many factors, such as the age of the animal, the nature of the problem, how long they have had it, and so on. An acute problem (short-term), like a minor accident, may take one or two treatments, whereas chronic (long-term) problems may take several treatments. Nature needs time to heal, and as long as treatment is having a positive effect, be patient and let it take its natural course.

Is it safe?

As mentioned before, McTimoney chiropractic is very gentle and has been adapted for use with animals. In trained hands it is perfectly safe and there are no adverse side effects. Your pet will not feel any pain or discomfort, since the practice applies gentle touch and no forceful adjustment is used. Your pet may feel far more discomfort by not being treated!

Case histories

'I've treated a lot of dogs for paralysis. One particular dog had fallen and twisted its neck and was totally paralysed. I also get a lot who are paralysed in their hind quarters and are totally incontinent.'
The Hon. Richard Arthur, McTimoney chiropractor

'Willie, a six-year-old Battersea bitsa dog, had been hit by a car some years earlier and his peculiar twisted back had always been noted but so far had not caused any problem. One day he collapsed completely, being unable to walk and in great pain and distress. Chiropractic treatment was sought. Willie was found to have considerable distortion in the pelvis with resultant misalignment in the lower lumbar vertebrae. Within 20 minutes of treatment he was able to get up and run about, to his owners' great joy. He made a complete recovery and went on to live for another ten years, enjoying his rabbiting in the countryside.'
Dana Green, McTimoney chiropractor

Useful information

Where to find a McTimoney chiropractor

As with other complementary treatments, the law prohibits anyone who is not a qualified vet from practising on animals. However, most chiropractors work closely with vets and have animals referred to them. If you wish to have chiropractic treatment for your pet then talk to your vet and get their approval. Most vets these days are happy to refer an animal to a qualified and experienced practitioner. If your vet does not know of a McTimoney chiropractor locally, you can contact the McTimoney Chiropractic Association. They will send you a directory of animal practitioners, all of whom are registered and licensed by the association.

The Administrator
McTimoney Chiropractic Association
21 High Street
Eynsham

Oxford OX8 1HE
Tel: 01865 880974
Fax: 01865 880975

CHAPTER NINE

Flower Essences

 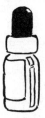

At-a-glance guide

What are they? Liquid drops of flower and plant essence.

What can they help? All sorts of emotional and behavioural problems, such as fear, loss, shock, anxiety and aggression.

Can you do it yourself? Yes. They are safe, easy to use and widely available.

Average cost of remedies? About the same as a two-and-a-half-kilo bag of brown rice.

Average cost of treatment? Generally less than standard veterinary fees, when seeing a registered flower remedy practitioner.

Flower essences work primarily on the emotional and mental levels of an animal and can help to restore health and harmony to its whole being. They make a great healing tool to use at home, especially since they are easy to use on pets, powerful yet harmless, and are relatively cheap!

Anyone who is closely involved with animals will know that they can experience stress just like us. They are sensitive to changes in their environment which, if adverse, can lead to behavioural problems or physical disease. The human–animal bond is a close one, and pets are particularly vulnerable to absorbing their owners' moods and emotions. Dogs and cats can experience fear, despondency, loneliness and depression just as we do, and they can pick up on our fears and frustrations. Flower essences have the power to heal negative emotions and make a powerful addition to your animal's health care.

The history of flower power

Flowers have been used for thousands of years throughout the world as one of many different natural healing traditions. Like herbs, they are one of the earliest forms of medicine. The healing property of flowers is nothing new, it is just that the knowledge of their curative power was temporarily lost, particularly in the Western world, where modern medicine took over from natural healing.

In Europe the use of flowers as natural remedies was 'rediscovered' and brought back into use by a British physician, Dr Edward Bach (1886–1936), who developed 38 different essences. His philosophy was 'A healthy mind ensures a healthy body', having found that once he had treated his patient's psychological state, their physical symptoms often disappeared too.

He enjoyed nature and observed how flowers could influence his mood, each different flower having a specific effect. While developing his remedies, he discovered that when he was in a particular state of mind or experiencing a particular emotion, certain plants and flowers could relieve that emotion. From this he developed his 38 remedies which he believed covered the whole range of human and animal emotions.

Although the most well-known flower essences are the Bach Flower Remedies, based on common British trees and plants like holly, impatiens and oak, nowadays there are many different ones emerging from all over the world. These include the Hawaiian Tropical Flower Essences, the Australian Bush Flower Essences and the Himalayan Flower Essences.

What are they?

Flower essences are a form of vibrational medicine. They work in a similar way to homoeopathic medicine in the sense that they are both an energetic imprint of the original substance. If you analysed the remedies scientifically you would not find a material amount of the original flower present. The energetic imprint of the original flower is transferred to water, which carries its healing energy.

How do they work?

Many forms of natural medicine are based on the belief that illness begins on emotional, mental or spiritual levels before it becomes apparent physically. For example, anger can manifest itself as a liver problem, mental rigidity can lead to arthritis, and grief can become cancer. Because of this, by healing the emotional state, the body can be completely cured. As animals are emotional beings and are just as affected by trauma, grief, loss or abuse as people are, and because they are so sensitive to subtle energies, the flower essences have a remarkable healing effect on them.

Animals also absorb a lot of stress from their owners. When we are stressed we stroke a cat, or we talk to our dog – and subconsciously they absorb our stress.

'Some people will say that they get on much better with their pets than anybody else! This is why we are so connected to our pets, especially to cats and dogs. The mere fact that they have nice soft coats that you can stroke calms our nervous system down.'
Clare Harvey, UK's leading authority on flower essences

Flower remedies act as a catalyst which boosts the animal's own powers of self-healing and balances its vital energy.

'I firmly believe that what sets flower essences apart from other forms of remedies is their ability to address physical, mental, emotional and spiritual aspects of the whole being to bring about a complete healing.'
Clare Harvey, UK's leading authority on flower essences

Flower essences work by bringing out positive emotions and getting rid of negative ones.

This is not like the effects of a mood-enhancing drug, which falsely changes an emotional state. Flower remedies work by unlocking inherent positive emotions and bringing them to the surface. For example, if you give an intolerant animal the beech flower remedy, this will help to bring about a tolerance of others from within the animal. Hornbeam will help a weak, despondent animal to find a renewed vitality and interest in its daily life.

'The remedies help us to feel ourselves again, at a point where we ceased to be quite ourselves.'
Dr Edward Bach

With animals, positive results can happen quickly because they are very direct in their emotions, thoughts and feelings about things, and so they can respond very quickly to essences. It is a simple and direct form of medicine for animals and helps them to becomes healthier and happier.

For an at-a-glance guide to the 38 Bach flower remedies traditionally used for certain emotional states, see over the page.

Rescue remedy is a unique combination of five Bach flower remedies: rock rose for terror, impatiens for impatience, clematis for dreaminess and lack of interest in the present, star of Bethlehem for the after-effects of shock, cherry plum for fear of the mind giving way.

What can be treated with flower remedies?
The most effective use for flower remedies is treating emotional and mental problems. They can reach deep into the animal's being and effect change at a very profound level – therefore all types of behavioural problems can be helped. Although flower essences primarily work on the emotional level, some of the essences also influence the physical body; these include hornbeam for giving strength, crab apple for clearing out toxins and olive for exhaustion. Some of the flower essences from other parts of the world also have very potent anti-viral and anti-bacterial properties.

FEAR

Terror	Rock Rose
Fear of known things	Mimulus
Fear of mind giving way	Cherry Plum
Fears and worries of unknown origin	Aspen
Fear or over-concern for others	Red Chestnut

OVER-CARE FOR THE WELFARE OF OTHERS

Selfishly possessive	Chicory
Over-enthusiasm	Vervain
Domineering, inflexible	Vine
Intolerance	Beech
Self-repression, self-denial	Rock Water

OVER-SENSITIVITY TO INFLUENCES AND IDEAS

Mental torment behind a brave face	Agrimony
Weak-willed and subservient	Centaury
Protection from change and outside influences	Walnut
Hatred, envy, jealousy	Holly

LONELINESS

Proud, aloof	Water Violet
Impatience	Impatiens
Self-centredness, self-concern	Heather

DESPONDENCY OR DESPAIR

Lack of confidence	Larch
Self-reproach, guilt	Pine
Overwhelmed by responsibility	Elm
Extreme mental anguish	Sweet Chestnut
After-effects of shock	Star of Bethlehem
Resentment	Willow
Exhausted but struggles on	Oak
Self-hatred, sense of uncleanliness	Crab Apple

UNCERTAINTY

Seeks advice and confirmation from others	Cerato
Indecision	Scleranthus
Discouragement, despondency	Gentian
Hopelessness and despair	Gorse
'Monday morning' feeling	Hornbeam
Uncertainty as to the correct path in life	Wild Oat

INSUFFICIENT INTEREST IN PRESENT CIRCUMSTANCES

Dreaminess, lack of interest in present	Clematis
Lives in past	Honeysuckle
Resignation, apathy	Wild Rose
Lack of energy	Olive
Unwanted mental arguments	White Chestnut
Deep gloom with no origin	Mustard
Failure to learn from past mistakes	Chestnut Bud

Some commonly treated problems include:

- Anxiety, fear

- Bereavement, loss, depression

- Aggression, jealousy, biting, scratching

- Hyperactivity, oversexed animals

- Stress, shock, trauma, accidents, during and after whelping

- Abuse, neglect

- Viruses

For specific ailments and first-aid use, see chapters 15 and 16.

Treating animals

Flower essences treat animals in an holistic way, treating the whole being, not just the symptoms of disease. With flower essences you can tailor-make a mixture of remedies or use just one at a time, depending on what is needed. If you do miss the mark there are no side effects, but it is always better to take your time and choose remedies that will best bring about positive changes.

By nature animals are highly sensitive and intuitive, and the remedies suit them very well. They are really no different from human beings in the sense that disease often begins on the emotional or mental level, and these have to be addressed before there can be a complete cure.

Remember, when you treat your animals, treat yourself at the same time. Animals really do mirror our emotions and that may be the root cause of their illness. By treating both the pet and its owner (and sometimes the whole household!), you usually get a more effective and long-lasting cure. If you have been through a stressful situation with your animal, like breaking up a dog fight, you may also benefit from taking one or more of the same remedies as your pet.

'You get a speedier healing of an animal if you can treat the owner at the same time. Often people bring me their animal for treatment and as their pet starts to get better they say, "Well, I will come along and have some too." That often happens, especially if there is a very close bond, when it is actually quite important to treat both the animal and the owner.'

Clare Harvey, UK's leading authority on flower essences

Case histories

'I usually recommend rescue remedy in situations involving the collapse of any young animal. It's a means of buying time. It's an excellent adjunct to any other treatment used for and during an immediate crisis. Try it; don't be concerned with [why or] how it works, since you might deprive yourself of a wonderful healing tool.'

J.G.C. Saxton, BVetMed, MRCVS (taken from *Rescue Remedy* by Gregory Vlamis, Thorsons, 1994)

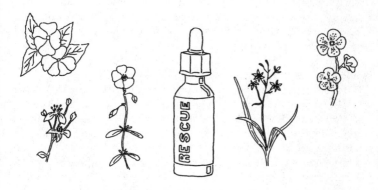

'A lady approached me for remedies for her two cats. Toc, a three-year-old female who had previously been treated with indifference and impatience by her first owners, was hyperactive and continually jumping on the older cat, who was frightened by Toc's behaviour. Mrs Green [the older cat] had always allowed herself to be pushed around by other cats, never standing up for herself, and her owner described her as a nervous cat, always holding back from strangers. Toc was given agrimony (for her restlessness), vervain (for her hyperactivity), impatiens (for her agitation, as she was always moving around at break-neck speed), beech (to allow her to be more tolerant of Mrs Green) and, finally, chicory (to address her "don't ignore me" behaviour towards the owner). Mrs Green was given larch (to boost her self-confidence), mimulus (to give her courage) and centaury (to allow her to be more assertive in the face of Toc's dominance). After a month, the owner wrote to say that Mrs Green was much bolder and not so nervous and had begun to stick up for herself against Toc. Toc was more tolerant towards Mrs Green and had stopped racing around the house at break-neck speed. She added that she had forgotten to mention that Mrs Green had been suffering from halitosis but does not have it any more and wondered if this could have been improved by the remedies as well!'

Christine Newman, registered Bach flower remedies practitioner

Choosing remedies for your pet

The main difference between animals and humans is that you cannot ask animals how they feel. However, you can observe their behaviour and characteristics and make an educated guess. If you know you have a nervous cat who has also experienced some kind of shock, you would give it remedies for shock and stress – maybe rescue remedy and aspen. It is a question of getting to know your pet and how they react to things.

It can really help if you put yourself in your pet's skin, so to speak. For example, if an animal has just been in a fight, imagine how you would feel after a fight – perhaps a mixture of shock, fear and generally feeling out of sorts? By doing this you can get a fair idea of what emotions the animal is going through. You might have a dog with a hurt leg who is trying to soldier on as if nothing was wrong – this might indicate an oak temperament where the animal is exhausted but struggles on regardless. Another dog might slink off into a corner and be irritable and snappy, which could indicate the need for willow to treat resentment.

A cat which is aloof by nature may become extra aloof when it is ill, and so you could give it water violet. This would be treating the animal's normal character as well as its specific reaction to the illness. Another cat which is normally aloof may become scared and anxious when ill, and so you could give it both water violet and aspen. When prescribing remedies for animals, their 'normal' temperament needs to be taken into account together with their specific mood. When an animal is ill, its mood will often change. Just like humans, animals may get very drowsy and lethargic and need clematis and wild rose, or they may seem unpredictable and snappy or scratchy and need something like holly.

Can you use several remedies at once?

You can use up to six remedies at the same time – but you need to make sure they complement each other, which is why it is important to spend time making a good diagnosis. You cannot do any harm by giving the wrong remedies – the animal's body just gets rid of them and there are no side effects – but it is better if you can be as accurate as possible in order to achieve a complete healing. Note that rescue remedy still counts as one remedy, even though it is already a mixture.

Flower essences provide a gentle, safe system of emotional stress relief.

Can they be used with other remedies and therapies?

You can use flower remedies at the same time as orthodox drug treatment, as they will speed up the healing process and help to clear out the drug side effects.

In general, the flower essences complement all forms of natural medicine very well and can be used either as a total system on their own or as part of a broader therapeutic treatment. Having said that, it is best not to mix flower essences with other energetic treatments, such as healing and homoeopathy, as they could interfere with each other. Let one energy medicine have a chance to restore the animal to health before bringing in another one. Some of the more physical therapies like nutrition, medical drugs, herbs or chiropractic, however, combine well with flower essences.

Using flower essences at home

Flower remedies really do lend themselves to home use because they are simple to use and easy to get hold of. There are hundreds of different essences from all over the world that can be used. Start by getting to grips with the Bach range, and then explore some of the other flower essences as you become more experienced and more knowledgeable.

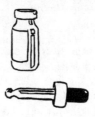

Dosage

The dosage is the same for cats and dogs as it is for people, usually three or four drops in their food or water. Drinking water should be fresh every day, so you need to remember to add more drops each time it is changed. Since cats do not drink a lot of water, put the drops in their food to ensure they are getting the remedy regularly.

Another way of giving it to cats and dogs is by putting it on their nose and allowing them to lick it off. Alternatively, you can put it on to their fur and it gets absorbed straight into their system.

Ideally the essences should be given three or four times a day. In cases of extreme stress they can be given every ten to twenty minutes until there is some relief.

When flower essences are given in food or water there is no need to worry about other pets in the house accidentally getting a dose too. They will not have any effect unless the animal is needing the same remedies – and the effects will be positive!

Length of treatment

There are no hard and fast rules, since complementary medicine is geared towards each individual animal. Pets with an acute condition, like shock, can be given a remedy every 15 minutes until they begin to calm. At the other end of the scale, when dealing with deeply ingrained emotional problems like the lingering effects of a past trauma, the healing process may take several months and the animal may only need three or four drops once a day.

Storing the flower essences

It is important to remember that the flower essences are liquid energy and can be influenced by other energies. It is particularly important to keep them away from any electrical appliances like televisions, computers, the mains electricity supply, and so on. Also keep them away from direct sunlight and strong smells such as essential oils and peppermint, as these can affect them. Like most medicines, if you store them in a cool, dry cupboard they should be fine. Correctly stored, flower essences will keep for at least five years.

Flower essences as preventative medicine

Flower essences work very well as preventative medicine because, caught early enough, stresses and strains on the emotional level can be prevented from later coming out as physical disease or behavioural problems. This is why it is good to have a bottle of rescue remedy handy, because whenever your pet experiences stress or has a shock, you can treat it immediately. An accident or fight can often be the trigger which weakens the body system, and the essences pull the system back together again. It is an invaluable remedy to have on tap as part of your first-aid kit for pets.

'I had one animal who had been in an accident and was obviously unconscious. He was given a couple of drops of rescue remedy and was immediately brought round into consciousness. It works that quickly with them.'
Clare Harvey, UK's leading authority on flower essences

Many vets use rescue remedy as a last resort after standard procedures have failed and have reported remarkable results.
(Taken from *Rescue Remedy* by Gregory Vlamis, Thorsons, 1994)

Using flower essences to help a dying animal

Flower essences can help the end of an animal's life to be much more bearable, whether it dies naturally or has to be put down by a vet. The essences can also help owners who are upset and distressed by watching a much-loved companion pass away. Flower essences can be used to make the last days more positive; they can help to make the situation less traumatic and can help you to be more accepting.

Bach flower remedy medicine chest for dogs

If you only have one flower essence in your medicine chest then make it the rescue remedy. You might be surprised how often you use it, not just for your pet, but for yourself too! However, if you are wanting to have a wider range of essences, the following is a list of some of the most commonly used Bach flower remedies for dogs and cats.

Aspen For the nervous, fearful dog, especially in new circumstances. This dog often has its tail between its legs, and may be a submissive wetter. Aspen can help dogs who have been harshly disciplined in the past.

Chestnut bud Helpful in training situations. Useful in teaching a puppy to make a distinction between right and wrong – for example, the difference between a rawhide bone and your shoes! Helps to break bad habits.

Chicory For a dog who follows you around, is constantly underfoot, and becomes extremely upset when left alone. For the jealous or possessive dog. For the affectionate dog who must always be in your lap.

Clematis Dogs will sometimes need clematis when kept indoors in stormy weather or when pining for their owner to come home. It can also be used if they are drowsy, but not really sleepy. It is useful following surgery to help them wake up after an anaesthetic. It may be used in combination with rescue remedy the moment puppies are born to help them wake up and breathe.

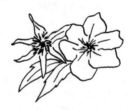

Holly For the angry dog who threatens attack, or attacks without provocation. Remember that any personality changes should be checked out with a vet. In addition, holly can be useful in treating aggressive behaviour often due to trauma or abuse in the past. (Use star of Bethlehem as well if there has been past trauma.)

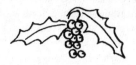

Honeysuckle For the dog whose owner or close companion has died or gone away. (Use it in conjunction with star of Bethlehem.) For the dog who acts withdrawn, subdued or unenthusiastic towards people. For homesickness while at kennels or if left alone for long periods of time.

Mimulus For a dog with a particular fear of known things, such as loud noises, thunderstorms, vacuum cleaners or small children. When these fears turn to terror, use rock rose or rescue remedy.

Olive For the dog who is totally exhausted from illness, hard work or trauma. This remedy may lend a measure of strength and comfort to seriously ill dogs when used with star of Bethlehem for physical or emotional trauma.

Rescue remedy Appropriate for any kind of accident, illness or injury your dog may experience. Can be used at dog shows, on car trips, while boarding, during a long absence, before or after surgery or whenever a dog seems to be experiencing the effects of extreme stress.

Scleranthus Can be useful in car sickness, used along with rescue remedy. Also good for seizures.

Star of Bethlehem For the physically or emotionally traumatised dog, either currently or in the past. Nearly always indicated for dogs who have been in a rescue centre or dog pound. For abused animals.

Vervain For highly strung, hyperactive dogs with a great deal of nervous energy. For those who are hard to stop from jumping up or barking. Where enthusiasm goes with the species, this remedy can help in slowing them down.

Water violet Useful for dogs who are aloof, self-reliant, intelligent

THE NATURAL WAY FOR DOGS AND CATS

and loners. Useful for dogs who were socialised comparatively late in life, and who seem very stand-offish. Often an excellent choice for dogs who have wild ancestry, such as the husky. It can be used for grieving animals who want solitude.

Bach flower remedy medicine chest for cats

These are some of the most commonly used remedies for cats.

Aspen For the fearful cat who is always slinking from safe place to safe place, never being quite at ease. For the cat who startles easily at any sound, even non-threatening sounds it has heard before.

Beech For picky eaters. For cats who have no tolerance for another animal or certain people. Effective with walnut to assist in keeping the peace between two cats who seem to be fighting. Good for jealous cats when a new person or animal joins the family.

Chicory For the extremely affectionate cat who can be possessive, jealous and always stays near you wanting to be held, petted and fussed over.

Clematis For use any time a cat appears stunned or experiences unusual patterns of sleeping beyond the typical cat-nap. Used in helping to regain consciousness after an accident or operation. Can be used in conjunction with rescue remedy to help newborn kittens wake up and breathe. One drop can be repeated every few minutes.

Honeysuckle For grief or homesickness. For the cat who has lost a person or other animal they have been close to. Star of Bethlehem can be used as well to address this condition. Also helpful along with walnut to help the cat adjust to a new location.

Hornbeam For fatigue. The strengthening remedy. Can be helpful in assisting runts or to build up any sickly animal.

Larch Especially useful for the low cat in the pecking order, perhaps the runt. For the cat with little or no self-confidence. Self-esteem is an important part of feline well-being and is usually radiated by an emotionally balanced cat.

Mimulus For fear of particular things or circumstances such as thunderstorms, vacuum cleaners or visits by small children. Where fear turns to terror, use rock rose or rescue remedy.

Rescue remedy Appropriate for any kind of accident, illness or injury your cat may experience. Can be used at cat shows, on car trips, while boarding, during a long absence, before or after surgery or whenever a cat seems to be experiencing the effects of extreme stress.

Star of Bethlehem For all trauma, past and present, physical and emotional. For recuperation from surgery, car trips, injury, boarding and other traumas that affect your cat's dignity, freedom, health or security. For cats adopted from shelters.

Vine For the boss cat who rules the roost and the household. Vine can make boss cats more tolerant of their companions.

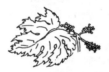

Walnut Very helpful for any changes that a cat may experience, such as new babies or new pets in the house, moving, weaning or heat cycles. It helps ease adjustment to holidays and changes to the normal routine.

Water violet A constitutional remedy for most cats which helps them keep their instinct for solitude in balance with enjoyable interaction with other animals and people. For aloof, loner animals. Good for grieving or sick animals who want solitude.

Useful information

Where to find a registered Bach flower remedy practitioner
Like most other forms of complementary medicine, the law prevents anyone who is not a vet from treating animals. However, many vets are happy to refer you to a qualified practitioner as long as they are kept informed about the treatment. If your vet does not know of a

practitioner who works with animals, then find someone yourself and ask your vet if they will refer your pet.

The Bach Centre (see below) will provide a list of registered practitioners in the UK who work with animals.

Where to buy flower essences

Bach Flower Remedies
The Edward Bach Centre
Mount Vernon
Sotwell
Wallingford
Oxon OX10 OPZ
Tel: 01491 834678 Fax: 01491 825022
E-mail: 101744.1312@compuserve.com

(For Bach flower essences, general advice, information, education, training, practitioners, newsletters, etc.)

The Bach flower remedies are widely available in health-food shops, chemists and some supermarkets.

The full range of international flower essences can be ordered from:
The Nutri Centre
7 Park Crescent
London W1N 3HE
Tel: 0171 436 5171

Further reading

The Encyclopaedia of Flower Remedies by Clare G. Harvey and Amanda Cochrane; Thorsons, 1995

Heal Thyself by Edward Bach; C.W. Daniel Co. Ltd, 1930; reprint 1990

Rescue Remedy by Gregory Vlamis; Thorsons, 1994

My Cat Is Driving Me Crazy! by Grace McHattie and Tim Couzens; Robinson

CHAPTER TEN

Healing

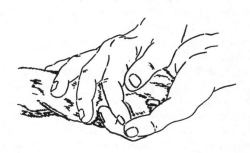

At-a-glance guide

What is it? Healing uses natural energy to stimulate an animal's own self-healing ability.

What will it help? Almost any condition, physical or behavioural, will benefit from healing.

Can you do it yourself? Yes. There are short courses on animal healing.

Average cost of treatment? Variable, but usually less than standard veterinary fees.

Most pets enjoy having healing treatment and know instinctively what it is and how it can help them.

Like most animals, dogs and cats are highly sensitive to energy. They seem to 'know' things before we do, and that is why we credit them with having a 'sixth sense'. It is this ability to tune into subtle influences that guides migratory birds across the world and lets animals know when there is a fierce storm brewing. Because healing is an energy medicine, it offers animals something natural which they immediately recognise in a way that most humans do not.

Animals have a highly developed sensitivity and they often pick up on our fears and anxieties. This is especially true for domestic pets, who soak up any negative emotions around the family home and often become ill or disturbed as a result.

How does it work?

Healing is simply the channelling of energy, or life force, through the healer into the animal. A healer acts as a link between this energy and the dog or cat, the energy usually being transmitted through their hands – hence the expression 'hands-on healing'.

It is a non-intrusive therapy, in the sense that nothing physical penetrates the body and no remedies are given. It is gentle and safe, yet very powerful.

Like other complementary therapies, healing treats the whole being, not just the disease symptoms. Without a harmonious balance between the mind, body and spirit, both people and animals eventually become ill. Because healing is such a profound therapy it can reach depths that many other types of medicine cannot.

Healing is one of the oldest forms of medicine in the world and was practised by all the ancient societies and cultures, from the Aborigines in Australia to the South-American Indians.

There are a variety of different healing methods that you may come across, including spiritual healing, Reiki, natural healing and crystal healing, all of which are essentially doing the same thing – using natural energy to restore health and well-being to an animal.

What is this healing energy?

It has many names, depending on individual understanding, beliefs and cultures. For example, in the West it is often called the life force, God force, nature or divine energy. The Chinese know it as 'chi' and in Indian medicine it is called 'prana'. However, the different names are less important than the understanding of what it is and where it comes from. Healers believe that this energy is all around us and within us and that it comes from one invisible intelligent source. It is the energy flow in all of life, and what animals are recognising is that they are a part of it, in the same way that plants and trees flow with the seasons and follow nature's infinite cycle of creation and decay.

Some people call this energy a love, a deep, unconditional love;

animals recognise this deep caring and how it can heal, in the same way that a child recognises that its mother's love can heal many of its hurts.

Healing animals

By tuning into the life force, the healer can transmit the healing energy to the animal. This helps to balance energy throughout the body, and stimulates the immune system, repairs tissues, revitalises an exhausted animal, calms distress, eases pain and gives an animal a greater sense of well-being.

Animals are very sensitive to healing energy and naturally understand it to the extent that they often offer the parts of them that are affected towards the healer's hands. For example, if there is something wrong with a cat's paw it might offer its paw, or if a dog has a pain in its stomach it might lie on its back and expose its stomach. They work with the healing energy and it almost becomes like a dance where the animal and the healer are working as a team.

In a way, healing is like jump-starting a car – it gives the animal's whole being a boost of energy and stimulates self-healing.

Which problems can healing help?

Healing can be effective for almost any illness as it is a truly holistic therapy. However, as with any natural treatment, every animal is an individual and will respond in different ways and to different degrees. The types of conditions that healers commonly treat include the following:

- Skin conditions, both long- and short-term

- Arthritis, rheumatism, musculo-skeletal problems

- Cancer (and other 'incurable' conditions)

- Behavioural problems such as nervousness or anxiety

- Pain relief

- Digestive problems

- Respiratory problems

- Trauma such as past abuse, maltreatment

Healing can be of real benefit to 'incurable' diseases, and although it may not effect a complete cure, it can improve the quality of your pet's life. Many people have observed that their animal is much happier and more content even though the illness is still there.

Where behavioural problems are concerned, pets often pick up on their owners' anxieties and then display behavioural problems as a result. For example, if their owner is frightened of being left alone or of being in the dark, the pet picks up on this anxiety and starts behaving differently. While the owner might not realise the extent of their own problem, they often see it in their pet and take the animal for healing. An experienced healer will notice what is happening and suggest the owner has healing too.

Behavioural problems may also stem from trauma, such as a fight with another dog or a frightening experience. Healing is especially useful for animals who have suffered a degree of abuse or neglect in the past. In the same way that you would take a 'rescued' cat or dog to the vet to have a check-up and its injections, healing helps pets to settle into a new home much more smoothly.

For specific ailments see chapter 16.

Why take your animal to a healer?

Healing is one of the most gentle and natural of therapies and can reach the very soul of an animal. It stimulates an animal's own powers of recovery and does not rely on any medicines or remedies. If you wish to try an alternative or complement to standard veterinary care, healing offers a powerful treatment. It is especially profound when dealing with behavioural problems and long-term conditions like eczema and arthritis, which traditional medicine often cannot help. Healing can improve the quality of life of a dying animal and can help that animal to go more peacefully when it is ready.

Sometimes a condition does not appear serious to the untrained eye, so it is vital to get a vet's diagnosis before deciding to seek complementary treatment. As long as the vet has seen your pet, a healer will be happy to see them too.

What to expect in a consultation

Some animals seem to sense the healing energy already in the room when they arrive for treatment and immediately become very still. It can be astonishing to witness the way that a really frisky animal will suddenly go still, lie down and become very quiet. Other animals might react in a completely different way, sniffing around the room as if trying to identify the energy before settling down.

During the consultation the healer may ask you questions about the nature of your pet's symptoms; for example, what diagnosis has been made, what medication it is on and what recommendations the vet has made, so as not to conflict with that advice. The healer may also ask about the animal's bowels, appetite, diet, sleeping and peculiar habits, if any, and offer advice on your pet's diet, perhaps recommending vitamin or mineral supplements.

During the actual healing, healers place their hands on or near to the animal and work over its body. How long is spent on each area will depend on how much that part needs; this is really an intuitive feeling on the healer's part. Some animals, especially cats, may not want to be touched at all, so healers place their hands close, but not actually touching the animal. If it is an aggressive animal, again they will heal at a distance. Healing is just as effective this way; however, most animals enjoy being touched. Something I often experience when healing cats who won't let me touch them is that when they come for a second healing it is as if they are a different cat and will let me place my hands anywhere without a fuss! They are recognising the healing and how it can help them.

On average, healing takes about ten to twenty minutes, but it really depends on the animal. A highly frisky dog like a bearded collie may take its healing quickly while on the run, whereas a more relaxed type of dog like a labrador may come in, lie down straight away and not move again until it has had its fill. In both cases the animal will be getting as much healing as it needs. Often animals let you know when they have had enough by getting up and wandering off.

Do animals enjoy healing?
Animals seem to enjoy healing and usually settle down to receive the treatment pretty quickly.

Healing is very soothing for an animal in pain or distress, and even healthy animals can benefit from regular healing to keep them well. I used to give regular healing at an animal sanctuary to a ewe who had a crippled back leg. Every time I began to give her healing some of the other animals, particularly the dogs, would try to nudge in to get a piece of the action! It got to the stage where I had to take the sheep into an enclosed pen so that I could keep all the other animals out while she received her treatment. This was definitely a case where animals were sensing the healing energy and wanted to have some themselves.

How many sessions will my pet need?

This is not something that you can predict, since it really depends on how well the animal absorbs the healing and what changes come about. A healer would be unlikely to recommend a specific number of treatments in advance; they are much more likely to decide after each appointment whether another one is needed, having assessed how the animal is getting on. Usually, however, you will notice some change after the first healing. A few of the most common things that people report is that their pet seems 'calmer', 'more peaceful' and 'more like itself'.

Is healing always about a cure?

Healing is not just about helping an animal to recover from illness or helping it to live well, it is also about helping it to die well. In my own practice I have given healing to several pets with terminal cancer whose vets cannot do any more for them. Usually their owners bring them for healing to help them to be as comfortable as possible for the time they do have left. Others are concerned that their pet dies in a dignified and peaceful way.

A healer will never influence anyone's decision on whether or not to have their pet put down; this decision has to be what the owner feels is right for them and for their animal. It can be a very traumatic experience to watch an animal losing its faculties, as anyone who has witnessed an ill pet will know. If you do decide to have your pet put down, healing can help them to go in peace.

Sometimes it seems as if an animal is hanging on to life when it really should have passed away. In cases like that a healer may explain how you can 'talk' to the animal about it, not necessarily outwardly but inwardly, and for a lot of people this really does help them to let their pet go. Time and again pets seem to wait for their owners to go away on holiday and then die while they are away. It is as if they are sparing them the experience of coping with their death. So there can be a need for 'talking' to the animal, and for saying inwardly, 'I love you, but I shall let you go to do whatever is right for you.'

Absent healing

Absent or distance healing is a way of giving healing to an animal without the healer actually being present. Healing energy can still be channelled to pets at a distance, sometimes transmitted via the owner.

Healing at home

Healing is a wonderful thing and comes naturally to a parent comforting an injured or sick child. In the same way, a loving touch and compassion for a sick or dying animal is very healing – and everyone is capable of doing that. However, if you would like to learn more about healing animals there are plenty of short courses you can go on which will give you an understanding of animal healing.

Healing as a first-aid/emergency measure

If a healer is present at an accident, a lot of good work can be done immediately. Healing helps to detraumatise the animal, relieve pain and bring it to a more peaceful state, which makes recovery easier.

When an animal has been involved in an accident it is vitally important it goes to the vet for a check-up, even if it looks like there is nothing wrong. It can have healing afterwards. If there are not any actual injuries, healing can help the animal to recover from the shock and reduce the trauma. If there are injuries then it will help to speed up the healing process in the tissues and bones. Be careful, though, not to cart a sick or injured animal around in the car too much. You could ask your healer to come to your home or to send absent or distant healing until you feel the animal is well enough to travel.

Can healing be used with other therapies?

Like other forms of complementary medicine, healing is a complete treatment on its own. It is therefore best not to use it simultaneously with similar therapies, such as flower remedies, acupuncture and homoeopathy, which also work with subtle energy. It does complement the more physical types of treatments, such as nutrition, chiropractic, osteopathy, herbal medicine and conventional veterinary treatment, and can help to enhance their effects.

Referrals from vets?

Healers try to work in harmony with vets, and more and more vets these days are becoming interested in complementary medicine and are happy to make referrals. Others may practise some form of natural treatment themselves; a lot of vets are taking training in natural medicine in order to incorporate it into their practice because they know of the profound effect it has on animals. Animal healing is no exception to this growth in complementary treatment for pets.

Case histories

'We had a six-month-old puppy here whose owners were told by the vet that nothing more could be done for it and that it had to be put to sleep. It was paralysed and couldn't move its legs, and had to be carried in on the first visit. On the second visit it walked in, and on the third it ran in! The owners said what difficulty they had restraining it from leaping about! That was lovely.

'We also had a cat who didn't purr. It was also always scared and anxious. When it came into the waiting-room it started to purr – for the very first time! What was happening was that the cat was picking up the caring, the love and the relaxation of the healing energy, so it felt able to "let go".'
Christy Casley, healer

No list of case histories would be complete without the story of my own dog, Basil. I got him aged about one from a rescue centre in Dorset, and as I was driving away with him in the back of the car I heard a faint voice in the distance shouting, 'He doesn't like being left alone.' Well, that proved to be an understatement! The first time I left him alone he ate the door frame around the back door in an attempt to get out. The second time I left him in my car for half an hour. When I returned he was in a high state of anxiety and had completely destroyed the inside of the car! There were teeth marks on the steering wheel, dashboard, safety belts and seat, and the head rests were in tatters. (The insurance company covered the repair costs of over six hundred pounds!) I immediately booked an appointment for him with a local healer. After just one healing it was like he became a different dog and he has never done anything like that again (he is now five). The power of healing never ceases to amaze me, and time and again I see animals responding in wonderful ways to this ancient art.

Useful information

How to find an animal healer

Most trained and qualified healers belong to a healing organisation (members are bound by a strict code of conduct in relation to treating animals) and can be contacted through them. You do not need a referral from a vet to take your pet to an animal healer, but it is always best to let your vet know what treatment your pet is having. Healers are not prevented by law from practising on animals in the same way that many other complementary practitioners are.

International Self-Realisation Healing Association
1 Hamlyn Road
Glastonbury
Somerset BA6 8HS
Tel: 01458 831353

ISRHA supplies a list of its animal-healer members in the UK.

National Federation of Spiritual Healers
Old Manor Farm Studio
Church Street
Sunbury-on-Thames
Middlesex TW16 6RG
Tel: 01932 783164

The NFSH supplies a list of its animal-healer members.

Training in animal healing

Self-Realisation Meditation Healing Centre
Laurel Lane
Queen Camel
Nr Yeovil
Somerset BA22 7NU
Tel: 01935 580266

Short courses in animal healing are open to anyone who wishes to learn about healing animals.

Further reading

Animals as Teachers and Healers by Susan Chernak McElroy; Rider Books

CHAPTER ELEVEN

Herbal Medicine

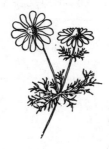

At-a-glance guide to herbal medicine

What is it? The use of plants to restore health and heal disease.

What can it help? Most physical problems, some behavioural problems.

Can you do it yourself? Yes.

Average cost of treatment? Home-grown herbs and those growing wild are free! Bought herbs are relatively inexpensive. Veterinary treatment using herbs will be in line with standard veterinary fees, possibly more expensive if it is a referral case.

Is it safe? Yes, when used sensibly and in the correct dosage.

Herbal medicine uses plants to heal. It is an holistic treatment and takes account of the animal's whole being and the many factors that unite to cause illness, such as inadequate diet and stress. Herbal medicine is gentle and often slow-acting but supports and stimulates the body to self-heal, so the results are long-lasting and potentially curative. Herbal medicine encompasses a range of well-

100

known plants, some of which we eat regularly, like parsley and mint.

Using plants to heal

Herbal medicine is one of the oldest forms of healing and, despite domestication, animals instinctively know which herbs and plants will help them when they are ill. How often have you watched your dog or cat eating grass and then being sick? If they are feeling ill they look for plants that will purge their system; at other times they may eat plants to get extra nutrients. Nature provides us with all we need; it is just a question of knowing what to take.

In the wild, animals usually eat the stomach contents of their prey first, because this is where the partially digested and highly nutritious plant material is. For the same reason, some dogs eat horse dung, especially when the grass is new, because they know it is a rich and digestible source of nutrients. I often watch my own dog pottering around in the garden picking out different plants and grasses – and he always eats horse dung in the spring!

Many vets and pet owners these days are rediscovering the power of herbs and, as a result, there are many different herbal remedies available – from fresh or dried herbs to tablets, ointments and tinctures.

How does it work?

Like other forms of natural medicine, herbs work in harmony with an animal's body and encourage it to self-heal and overcome illness. Because it is such an ancient form of medicine, the therapeutic plants are well documented and most herbal remedies are used in low doses with side effects rare.

Herbs contain a range of active constituents which help the body fight unwanted ailments. For example, they can sedate overactive organs, relax tense muscles and nerves, stimulate circulation, strengthen tissues, revitalise the body, boost the immune system and reduce inflammation. Essentially, herbs support the body systems in fighting disease, rather than just relieving the symptoms.

'Mammalian bodies are designed to live a healthy life – this is their natural state, this is their birthright – and the body has a tendency to make efforts to return to being healthy. So when you are looking at things holistically you are attempting to help the body to return to

being healthy. You are also trying to remove the influences – medicinal, nutritional or environmental – which are harmful and which lead to ill health.'
John A. Rohrbach, MVetMed, MRCVS

Using herbs with animals

In most cases the same herbs that are used for treating humans can also be used safely for dogs and cats, with a few exceptions. Cats are highly sensitive to some herbs and often react differently from dogs. The herbs not to give cats are marigold, marijuana, cocoa or white willow bark. However, when in doubt check with your vet or a herbalist and stick to the commonly used herbs until you get more experienced.

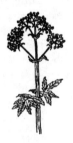

Plants contain natural healing powers, and because of their long history we know which plants we can use safely and what effect they will have. For example, skullcap and valerian are commonly used for treating nervous problems in animals as they have a calming and soothing effect, and psyllium husks are great for alleviating constipation. An example of some old herbal remedies for treating burns I came across in *Animal Cures the Country Way* by Robin Page is to use a raw potato or honey and vinegar.

It is easy to forget that before modern medicine, herbal medicine was an everyday way to cure ills. Because of the popularity of fast-acting modern drugs, herbal medicine has taken a back seat, but as more and more people are concerned with the side effects of drugs and are wanting more natural treatments for themselves and their pets, herbal medicine is enjoying a great revival.

Can herbs be harmful?

Not everything that is natural is necessarily safe, and some herbs are toxic in large doses. Just because the side effects are minimal and instances of adverse reactions are rare, it does not mean that herbal medicines are completely safe to take. Herbs are powerful medicines and need to be treated with respect. Anything taken in excess or taken inappropriately may be detrimental.

Something you have to be careful of in herbal medicine is getting a diagnosis and then treating your animal yourself without veterinary supervision. Talk to your vet and say you want to try something other than drugs; most vets will be happy to refer you as long as they can keep their eye on the situation. You have to play safe with difficult conditions, but anything that is not life-threatening you can treat yourself with herbs. The answer is not to give anything if you do not know what it is or what it is expected to do.

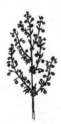

Healing properties of herbs

Herbal medicine covers a vast range of healing possibilities, from the mild-acting plant medicines like chamomile and peppermint to the very potent ones like pokeroot and wormwood. Herbs have different properties, ranging from nutritive to medicinal.

Herbs are easy to get hold of and come in many forms – fresh herbs, dried, tinctures, tablets, ointments, compresses, poultices, infusions, decoctions, oils and capsules – and there are several herbal remedies specifically made for dogs and cats (see suppliers at end of chapter).

What can herbal medicine help?

It can help most physical illnesses and disorders, such as chronic, long-term problems like arthritis and rheumatism, and some of the more acute problems like kennel cough and other bacterial infections. Herbal remedies can also help with behavioural problems, such as anxiety and nervousness. Below is a guide to some of the conditions herbal medicine is effective in treating:

- Rheumatism, arthritis

- Skin problems, such as eczema

- Digestive problems, such as diarrhoea, constipation, colic, wind

- Infections

- Worms, parasites, fleas

- Kidney conditions

- Respiratory problems

- Heart problems

- Nervous conditions

Herbal medicines can also be used for a wide range of minor problems that are easy to treat at home, including stomach upsets, vomiting, constipation, diarrhoea, digestive problems, sore muscles, skin rashes, burns and allergies.

Properly used, herbs can have a gentle action and help the body to heal itself.

For specific ailments, see chapter 16.
For first-aid use, see chapter 15.

Consulting a herbal vet
If you wish to use herbal treatment for your pet but the case is too

complicated or too serious to treat safely at home, get a referral to a vet who uses herbal treatments in their practice (see further information at the end of the chapter).

'It is very important that if people do not want orthodox treatment and instead want herbal treatment, they should say so to their vet. I have some vets who ask me to treat their own animals, and some of them have come to thinking in this way because again and again they are hearing from clients who are interested in using herbs and they think there might be something in this.'
John A. Rohrbach, MVetMed, MRCVS

Selecting the right herbs for the problem can have a profound healing effect without the danger of side effects associated with many modern drugs.

'There are a variety of reasons why people ask me for herbal treatment for their pets. Some regard it as a natural form of medicine to be used. Others want to avoid continued orthodox treatment – repeated courses of antibiotics, steroids yet again – or even to avoid an operation. Some people have a knowledge of what herbs can do and they want it because they know it is a very effective form of treatment.'
John A. Rohrbach, MVetMed, MRCVS

The healing action of herbs
Herbs are often categorised according to the kind of problem they will help. The right herb can be chosen by knowing what effect it will have on the body and what effect you are wanting.

Below is a list of some of the actions herbs have which make them beneficial for healing disease:

- Anthelminitic herbs destroy or expel intestinal worms, e.g. wormwood, garlic.

- Bitter herbs have a special role in preventative medicine and stimulate appetite, aid the liver in detoxification and stimulate gut-healing, e.g. wormwood, barberry.

- Carminative herbs stimulate the digestive system and soothe the gut wall. They reduce any inflammation, ease griping pains and help to get rid of gas in the digestive tract, e.g. ginger, peppermint.

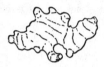

- Demulcent herbs soothe and protect irritated or inflamed tissue, especially in the bowel. They help prevent diarrhoea and reduce the muscle spasms that cause colic, e.g. slippery elm.

- Laxative herbs promote bowel movement, e.g. cascara, aloe vera.

- Nervine herbs help to strengthen and tone the nervous system. Some act as stimulants and some as relaxants, e.g. skullcap and valerian.

- Vulnerary herbs are applied externally and help to heal wounds and cuts, e.g. aloe vera, comfrey.

Treating your pet with herbs at home

One of the best uses for herbs is as a preventative measure – *before* health problems appear. Because they strengthen and tone, herbs can be part of your pet's natural diet throughout their life and can help to keep them healthy and strong.

There may be times when you need to use fast-acting medical drugs, but when there is no danger to the animal, herbs make powerful healing agents. In many of the chronic cases, such as arthritis, herbs can often replace drugs entirely, although reduction of medication should only be carried out under the supervision of a vet. Many people prefer using whole plant remedies to avoid any adverse side effects that may be found with modern drugs.

Herbal medicine is also helpful in day-to-day first-aid treatment for things like cuts, burns and bites. Any first-aid treatment should be short-lived. If there is no improvement fairly quickly, then take your pet to the vet.

Keep in mind the fact that although herbs are gentle and safe, they are medicines and should be treated with respect. Always stick to the tried and tested remedies, or consult a herbal vet for more complicated cases. When buying herbs always make sure they are from a reputable source, since the quality of the herbs used will determine their therapeutic potential. Only use high-quality herbs/herbal preparations or you will not get the healing effects that you wish.

Cost and availability
Freshly picked herbs cost nothing and you can grow your own. However, this is not always possible, and herbs and herbal products are relatively cheap and come in many forms. They are readily available in health-food shops, chemists and herbalists or by mail order (see stockists at end of chapter).

How to use herbs for healing
Herbs can be taken internally or used locally on wounds. They make great first-aid remedies – within half an hour they can be boiled up and ready to use as a poultice or compress. If you have ointments, tinctures, pills or capsules to hand, they can be used immediately.

One of the easiest ways to use herbal treatment is to get the ready-prepared ones for dogs and cats which come in tablets, tinctures and lotions. They always have instructions for use, which makes them a good starting point until you feel ready to branch out and prepare your own. Once you feel more confident about using herbs for healing it is fun to collect and prepare them yourself, and you will get great joy and satisfaction finding out more about herbal medicine and harvesting nature's healing garden.

Preparing your own herbs
You can either grow your own in the garden or in pots on a windowsill, or gather herbs growing wild, such as nettles and dandelions. Try not to pick herbs that are growing too near a road, as these will be polluted. Freshly picked herbs should be used fairly soon after picking or frozen for later use. Dried herbs will last for about a year as long as they are completely dry before storing. The

best way to store dried herbs is in a dark glass jar or in a brown paper bag, keeping them in a cool, dark place.

Freshly picked herbs These can be chopped up and put straight into your pet's food, e.g. parsley, garlic, dandelion.

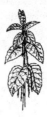

Dried herbs These can be sprinkled on food, e.g. nettle, comfrey, echinacea, or made into a tea. Dried herbs can also be ground into a powder using a coffee grinder or herb grinder.

Infusion or tea You can make a tea from plant leaves and small stems by soaking one teaspoon of dried herbs (or two teaspoons of fresh herbs) in a cup of boiling water and leaving it for 20–30 minutes. The strained liquid will keep in the fridge for a few days. This is a good way of using common garden herbs like nettles, parsley and dandelions. Always use distilled or filtered water. The correct dosage of herb tea can be mixed into your pet's food or given in a dropper bottle straight into their mouth. Tilt their head back a little so that the liquid runs down their throat.

Decoction This is a tea made from roots, bark, stems or seeds. Put one rounded teaspoon (or three for fresh herbs) of the crushed or chopped herb into water and simmer gently for about 30 minutes. Leave it to cool, strain and use as an infusion. This will last a few days in the fridge. Always use distilled or filtered water and a non-aluminium pan. This can be given in the same way as a herb tea.

Capsules These contain powdered herbs and can be given with or without food, depending on how your pet reacts. Pets often don't like taking capsules, so you can tip the contents into their food.

Tablets Powdered herbs. These can be taken with or without food and crushed to make them easier to take.

Tinctures Herbs that have been preserved in alcohol or some other preserving agent are called tinctures. They come in dropper bottles and can easily be dropped into an animal's mouth or into their food. Tinctures are easy to use and they last for several years without losing their potency. It is best not to use tinctures preserved in alcohol when treating pets with any kind of liver disease.

External use
Ointments Herbal ointments such as calendula and comfrey are good for external use on cuts and wounds.

Poultice A poultice of fresh herbs can be useful in a first-aid situation. To make a poultice, mash fresh plants with a little boiling water to make a paste. This can be placed on the affected area when still hot, but not boiling, and covered with a piece of gauze.

Compress These can be used hot or cold. A hot compress helps to bring heat to the area in order to kill germs, stimulate drainage and relax muscles. Soak a clean cloth in a herbal tea and apply hot (not boiling) to the infected area. Cover it with a dry towel to keep the heat in. After five minutes refresh the compress and reapply. You can do this for 15 minutes if your pet will let you, twice a day for up to two weeks. Hot and cold compresses can be alternated to stimulate blood supply to the area.

Soaking Make a warm infusion and immerse the animal's leg, tail or foot in the liquid for at least five minutes before drying. This can be done twice a day for up to two weeks.

Powders Goldenseal powder for infections and cuts; witch hazel to stop bleeding of minor wounds.

Length of treatment
It really depends on what is being treated. For example, an acute, short-term condition like diarrhoea can respond very quickly, whereas a longer-term chronic condition like arthritis can take much longer to respond. In general, allow only a day for an acute illness and

THE NATURAL WAY FOR DOGS AND CATS

two to three weeks for chronic things before any great improvement can be seen. When in doubt consult your vet or a medical herbalist.

Dosage

It is important to give the correct dosage. Using more than the suggested dosage does not mean better results.

Cats and small dogs ¼ teaspoon of an infusion or decoction three times a day, or two drops of tincture. Tiny pinch of dried herbs or half a teaspoon of fresh herbs.

Medium dogs ½ teaspoon of an infusion or decoction three times a day, or five drops of tincture. A pinch of dried herbs or ¾ teaspoon of fresh herbs.

Large dogs 1–2 teaspoons of infusion or decoction three times a day, or nine drops of tincture. ½ teaspoon of dried herbs or one teaspoon of fresh herbs.

This can be given until the symptoms disappear, or for a maximum of a week. If there is still no improvement, consult your vet. The capsules and tablets made specifically for dogs and cats have instructions for use on the container. When using your own herbs fresh or dried, they can be mixed into your pet's food.

For chronic conditions, use the same dosage as above but continue for eight to twelve weeks.

Response to treatment

The action of herbal treatment can be so gentle that you may think nothing is happening, but be patient and watch your pet carefully so that you notice any changes, as these will help you to decide what effect treatment is having and whether to continue it, stop it or try something else.

One of the first signs that natural treatments are working is that the animal seems 'more like itself', with better energy and a better mood. Physical improvements can often be slower to occur, so be aware of possible psychological changes. Sometimes there may be a healing reaction, such as a discharge, which is another sign that healing is taking place. A healing reaction is usually short-lived but if you are in any doubt as to whether your animal is getting worse, call the vet. It can take time for poisons to be eliminated from an animal's system and for strength and vitality to return.

Herbal medicine chest for cats and dogs

Aloe vera – Healing agent. Taken internally (liquid) and externally (gel or spray). Good for burns, cuts, wounds, insect bites and skin irritations. Used internally for a range of digestive complaints, as a general tonic and for its cleansing properties.

Comfrey – Healing agent. As a cream. Good for bruises, cuts and wounds. Helps to heal bones.

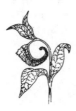

Distilled witch hazel Reduces inflammation and irritation; protects against infection. Good for wounds and burns. Can also be used powdered or as a cream.

Echinacea Fights infections; boosts the immune system. Commonly available as capsules, dried herbs and tablets.

Eye bright Eye problems. Can be take internally or used externally (tea) as an eye wipe.

Garlic Antiseptic, anti-fungal, anti-viral and anti-bacterial properties. Effective in treating parasites and infections. Helps to boost the immune system. Best used fresh or in capsule form if your pet does not like the taste of fresh garlic.

Ginger Soothing to the digestive system. Good for indigestion and wind. Also a warming herb and helps circulation problems and arthritis. Helpful for relieving travel sickness. Commonly used as capsules.

Psyllium husks For cleansing the bowel, detox of bowel. Used as capsules or loose.

Slippery elm Soothing. Good for digestive problems and stomach pains. Tablets or powder.

Herbs in the diet

Small quantities of ordinary culinary herbs like thyme, marjoram, sage, rosemary, parsley, dandelion, nettle and watercress are useful additions to the diet. They have health-giving properties in themselves and are good sources of minerals, vitamins and trace elements. Nettles, for example, are rich in vitamin C and iron, parsley is high in vitamin C, and kelp contains a wide range of essential elements. You can mix a few herbs together in a container and sprinkle a small pinch of the mixed herbs on your pet's food a few times a week. Cats and dogs will naturally go out and chew on herbs – it is all part of a good, healthy, balanced diet.

Herbal medicine has a place in modern veterinary practice and is regaining its traditional place in many surgeries for the treatment of common and chronic complaints.

Can herbs be given at the same time as other medicines?

In general they can be given along with standard veterinary treatment and some of the complementary treatments like acupuncture and chiropractic. However, some people would advise against giving strong-smelling herbs like garlic and peppermint at the same time as homoeopathic remedies or flower remedies, since the herbs can affect these and cause them to lose their potency. It is usually a good idea to give one type of natural treatment a chance to work before adding another one.

Case history: a cat with fleas and an allergy to flea bites

'Ferdinand is a large tabby and white cat. He was infested with fleas. In addition he had the typical scabby skin lesions that result from an allergy to flea bites. His owner had been taking him to the local vet for treatment, and she had been supplied with two toxic chemical sprays: one to use on Ferdie and the other to be sprayed around the house. In addition the vet had been treating him with corticosteroids to reduce the symptoms of allergy. Ferdie's owner did not think this was the best, or indeed the safest, course of action, either for Ferdie or for the human inhabitants of the house.

'She asked for a referral to this practice for herbal treatment. With a problem like this it was necessary to do more than simply use a herbal medicine; a more holistic approach was necessary. So other treatment and measures were advised in additon to the herbal treatment.

'Herbal treatment was sent in the form of a liquid medicine to be given by mouth. This consisted of extracts in diluted glycerin of: burdock root (*arctium lappa*), yellow dock root (*rumex crispus*), chebulic myrobalan fruit (*terminalia chebula*), emblic myrobalan fruit (*emblica officinalis*), liquorice root (*glycyrrhiza glabra*), fenugreek seed (*trigonella foenum-graecum*) and southernwood leaf (*artemisia abrotanum*).

'The treatment with corticosteroids had only been intermittent and the cat had not had any for several weeks, so it was not necessary to arrange for a gradual reduction in the dosage of this medication. (If treatment with corticosteroids has been given at sufficient dosage over a period of time the patient's adrenal glands atrophy, with the result that their ability to produce the natural hormones is reduced. Sudden cessation of treatment in this situation could put the patient at risk of a life-threatening illness, particularly if any other condition or accident occurred in the ensuing weeks.)

'Dietary supplements of capsules containing natural vitamin E and capsules of evening primrose oil and fish oil were supplied. His diet was improved by ceasing dry food and a poor-quality tinned food; he was instead fed tinned food made by a reputable manufacturer. Later, some cooked mashed vegetables were added to this.

'Advice was given about how to reduce the reinfestation from hatching fleas in the house by vacuum-cleaning. In view of the tender and irritated state of his skin, no medication was used against fleas; however, he was groomed gently once daily and attempts were to be made to catch and kill any fleas that could be found.

'A few weeks later a very dilute suspension of tea tree oil was supplied. This was sprinkled over the coat before grooming. Soon there was a reduction in the intensity and amount of skin licking and scratching that Ferdie was doing; the scabs disappeared and his fur started to grow.

'In subsequent years his owner has phoned when the symptoms reappear. The same treatment, but without the tea tree oil, has been sent and within two weeks he has improved.'
© 1997 John A. Rohrbach, MVetMed, MRCVS

Useful information

Where to find a herbal vet
The Hon. Secretary
The British Association of Homoeopathic Veterinary Surgeons
Chinham House
Stanford-in-the-Vale
Faringdon
Oxon SN7 8NQ
Ask for names and addresses of vets using herbal remedies.

John A. Rohrbach
MVetMed, MRCVS
Ard-Laggan
Perth Road
Crieff
Perthshire PH7 3EQ
Tel: 017646 53320

Suppliers of herbal products for cats and dogs
Hilton Herbs Ltd
Downclose Farm
North Perrott
Crewkerne
Somerset TA18 7SH
Tel: 01460 78300
Fax: 01460 78302

Dorwest Herbs
Shipton Gorge
Bridport
Dorset DT6 4LP
Tel: 01308 897272
Fax: 01308 897929
E-mail: dorwest@cix.compulink.co.uk

Denes Natural Pet Care
2 Osmond Road
Hove
East Sussex BN3 1TE
Tel: 01273 325364 (free advisory service)

Napiers Mail Order
Forest Bank
Barr
Ayrshire KA26 9NT
Tel: 01465 861625

Herbs of Grace
5 Turnpike Road
Red Lodge
Bury St Edmunds IP28 8JZ
Tel: 01638 750140

Further reading

The New Natural Cat by Anitra Frazier; Plume (Penguin), 1990
The Complete Herbal Handbook for the Dog and Cat by Juliette de
 Bairacli Levy; Faber and Faber, 1991
The Natural Remedy Book for Dogs and Cats by Diane Stein; The
 Crossing Press, 1994
The New Holistic Herbal by David Hoffman; Element Books, 1990

CHAPTER TWELVE

Homoeopathy

At-a-glance guide
What is it? Minute doses of natural substances usually given in tablet form. Works on the principle of 'like cures like'.
What can it help? Most physical diseases, mental and emotional problems, injuries and bruising.
Can you do it yourself? Yes.
Average cost of the remedies? The remedies are relatively inexpensive, and are widely available.
Average cost per treatment by a homoeopathic vet? In line with standard veterinary fees. However, the extra time involved can mean it is more expensive, in line with referral fees.

Homoeopathy is one of the most popular complementary treatments for animals and many vets through Britain use it in their practice. It lends itself particularly well to home use since the remedies are simple to use, easy to get hold of and inexpensive.

Homoeopathy is an holistic treatment and treats each animal as an individual. It is just as effective on cats and dogs as it is with people and they generally respond well, disproving any claims of a placebo effect. It is a gentle treatment for animals and allows them to heal from the inside out.

How it began

Although the 'similia principle' (like cures like) dates back to hundreds of years BC it was only rediscovered about 200 years ago by a German doctor, Samuel Hahnemann, who went on to build up a repertoire of diseases and remedies. While conventional medicine treats illness with an antidote, homoeopathy treats illness with a similar substance, only potentised. Hahnemann developed the potentising of natural substances to avoid harmful side effects. He also discovered that homoeopathy treats the whole being and works just as well with emotional and mental problems as it does with physical disease.

How does it work?

Homoeopathy is an energy medicine, and just like the flower essences, acupuncture and healing it has a positive effect on the animal's vital force. Homoeopathy sees symptoms of disease as a disturbance of the vital force and therefore by positively stimulating it, the animal's own powers of self-healing are set in motion.

Homoeopathy works on the principle of 'like cures like' in the sense that a substance that can cause symptoms of illness can also be used in a potentised form to treat those symptoms. For example, a fever similar to belladonna poisoning could be cured by potentised belladonna.

Like the flower essences, homoeopathic remedies do not contain any material or physical amount of the original substance. The substance is diluted over and over again until only its energy or vibration is left. The more diluted it is, the more far-reaching is its healing potential.

Homoeopathy does not treat the disease, it treats the animal with the disease.

Using homoeopathy with animals

One of the biggest moving forces behind bringing homoeopathy into modern veterinary use was the late George MacLeod, who wrote numerous books on treating animals with homoeopathy, from goats and horses to cats and dogs. Since the 1980s there has been a recognised training in veterinary homoeopathy and nowadays it is the most widely used natural medicine for treating animals. Because is it harmless and simple to use it has also become one of the most popular remedies to use at home.

Making a diagnosis

The key to successful treatment lies in getting the right match for the animal's symptoms with the properties of the remedy. When building a 'picture' of the disease, homoeopathy takes account of:

- The actual signs or symptoms, which might be diarrhoea, sickness and lethargy

- The length of time the animal has been ill

- The general constitutional type of the animal (for example, a labrador is prone to being slow and fat, whereas a setter is bouncy and lively)

- The individual characteristics of the animal

- The modalities – better or worse when hot or cold, better or worse with movement

- Odd characteristics, such as a fever but no thirst

Once you have a 'disease picture' you can choose the right homoeopathic remedy. When treating less complicated cases this is fairly easy to do and many of the remedies suit particular symptoms, such as arnica for bruising or aconite for shock. In cases like this the diagnosis is simple, and very often you will be able to treat your cat or dog effectively yourself and recovery can be rapid. Sometimes, though, the situation may be too complicated to manage by yourself, and with these cases it is best to seek the advice of an experienced homoeopathic vet (see 'Where to find a homoeopathic vet' at the end of the chapter).

'It is not always easy to see the true picture. In general, the more drug treatment an animal has had the more confused the picture of disease is. Homoeopathy often works stage by stage, like peeling the layers off an onion. You treat the symptoms you see to start with, and as the symptoms change, the animal is still ill, but you treat the new picture. You're peeling back layers of the onion until you get to the essential problem, and it can take time to get to the heart of it.'
June Third-Carter, VetMFHom

Consulting a homoeopathic vet

There are many vets who practise homoeopathy, and details of how to find one are given at the end of the chapter.

Appointments can take up to half an hour, during which the homoeopath will want to amass as much information as possible about the animal in order to build up a picture of the disease.

Healing reactions

Homoeopathic remedies stimulate and support the body's own healing mechanism and sometimes this leads to an 'aggravation' or flare-up of symptoms. If a remedy is spot-on and fits the picture accurately, the animal can get a brief increase in the severity of the symptoms. An itchy rash will become a horrendously itchy rash, and an animal suffering from a digestive problem may get a bout of diarrhoea. In homoeopathy this is seen as a good sign, because it shows that the remedy is working and that the animal's natural forces of recovery are in action. Healing reactions like these are usually quick to pass, but if severe must be relieved. It is not fair to expect an animal to suffer a bad reaction.

'I believe homoeopathy is a purer form of medicine than allopathy, but both have their uses.'
June Third-Carter, VetMFHom

The remedies

The remedies come from plant, animal or mineral sources, such as poppies, toad poison and oyster shells. They are made by qualified pharmacists and are produced by diluting the original substance in water or alcohol often thousands of times and shaking it vigorously to release its curative energy. This process makes even poisonous substances perfectly safe to use.

The remedies are made in different potencies or dilutions. The potencies are always indicated on the container and come in dilutions of tens, hundreds or thousands. A ten-times dilution is marked with an x, a hundred-times dilution is marked with a c, and a thousand-times dilution is marked with an m. With animals you will usually be using lower potencies of 6c or 30c, and these are the ones you will find in chemists and health-food shops.

High or low potencies are not stronger or weaker in the normal sense, but more like different radio frequencies – a low potency carries a wide range and will help even if it is not spot-on. A high potency carries a much narrower range so that it must be spot-on to have an effect – and the effect can last for months or years.

Remedies are usually sold in tablet form, as tiny sugar milk pellets which can easily be crushed and placed on an animal's tongue. Other forms of homoeopathic medicine include ointments, tinctures, powders and creams.

Are they safe?
For first-aid use in the low potencies the remedies are perfectly safe and you cannot give an overdose. Quantity makes no difference to the overall effect. Whether you take 100 tablets or one tablet, the effect will be the same. If it is the right remedy the effect will be positive; if it is the wrong remedy nothing will happen. Giving more than the required dose is just a waste, since it won't have an enhanced effect.

With very deep-seated or long-term ailments, prolonged use of the wrong remedy can muddy the picture or stall the healing process, so consult a homoeopath first.

What can it help?
Because homoeopathy is an holistic treatment and treats the whole being, it can have a therapeutic effect on almost any problem as long as the right remedy is used. You could say that homoeopathy works well for almost any condition, but not for every animal. When an animal does not respond to a remedy there can be a number of reasons why, including the wrong remedy having been given or the picture being muddled by a history of drug treatment or a strong family history of a problem.

Minor, short-term acute problems respond well. These include diarrhoea, constipation, bee stings, bruising, allergies and vomiting.

Chronic, long-term conditions which respond well include skin problems, arthritis, diabetes, emotional disorders and epilepsy.

In homoeopathy, treat the individual animal and it will fight the disease itself.

For specific ailments, see chapter 16.
For first-aid use, see chapter 15.

Case histories

'A good example of how quickly a remedy can work is the case of a collapsed dog that I went out to see on a house call. The dog was cold and its pulse was weak. I gave it aconite and by the time I had driven back to the surgery it was up on its feet – a good illustration of giving aconite for shock.'

'I had a dog with a skin problem that was really stumping me until I got his mother brought in. She always had skin trouble and I was able to see a clearer "picture" with her, and got the remedy that way. I just couldn't get it from seeing him, but I got it from seeing the mother's constitution. Long-term things like that which come through the generations often can't be cured, but they can be eased.'

'Ginger was a 14-year-old cat with liver failure who came to see me. He was emaciated, jaundiced, off his food and had a very swollen liver. With a mixture of phosphorus and ptelea he regained his appetite within 48 hours and steadily recovered over a month, having no further problems. Before this he was on antibiotics and steroids and he had been deteriorating rapidly.'
June Third-Carter, VetMFHom

Advantages of treating an animal homoeopathically

As with other forms of natural medicine, by treating your pet with homoeopathy you have the chance of getting a complete cure because it is getting to the root cause of the problem and leaving the animal stronger afterwards. A long course of antibiotics or steroids, by contrast, will leave the animal weakened. Although modern drugs relieve pain and stop infections, they also have side effects. In the end they leave the animal in a weaker position and so there is more likely to be trouble in the future, but you may get the animal through a crisis.

Home use

There are thousands of different homoeopathic remedies, but don't panic – you won't have to get familiar with them all! Certain remedies work for a variety of common complaints and make up a good all-round medicine chest to use at home. Always seek veterinary help in serious cases or if your animal is suffering a lot of pain.

All homoeopathic remedies have Latin names but are best known by their abbreviated versions. For example, calcarea carbonica is known as calc. carb. and rhus toxicodendron is known as rhus tox.

There are several very good books on homoeopathy for animals which will give you further insights into using this form of natural medicine. (see 'Further reading').

Buying the remedies

Each remedy is clearly labelled and will have its abbreviated Latin name marked on the container, along with its strength or potency (see the end of the chapter for stockists). They come in tiny sugar milk tablets which are easy for animals to take, and some companies make soft tablets specially for animals.

The remedies come in a range of different potencies, but when treating animals 6c strength is the best one to use. A homoeopathic vet may well use much stronger remedies, but unless you are experienced it is best to stick to 6c or 30c with your own pet.

Dosage

The amount given for cats and dogs is the same as for people, since size is not an important factor. The frequency of the dose is very important and depends on whether the disease is chronic or acute.

In urgent, acute cases

Give one tablet every 15 to 20 minutes for the first three hours, then one tablet every hour for the rest of the day. After that give one tablet three times a day for a few more days or until the symptoms have disappeared.

If it is something that is very severe, give the remedy and if you are not getting an improvement in an hour or two go to the vet. In less severe cases, if there is no change at all within 24 hours you could try a different remedy. It is important to watch your pet's reaction after they take the remedy, since any change is a sign that healing is taking place. Often they will become very relaxed and go to sleep.

Do not keep trying different remedies; if your pet does not respond to one or two in the first few days then seek professional help. Common sense must be applied when dealing with acute cases.

In chronic cases

Give one tablet three times a day for a week, then one tablet twice a day for another few weeks. If the problem is very long-term then one tablet a week for several weeks will be enough. Often results can come long after the remedy has been given and, as a rule of thumb, the longer a condition has been around the longer it will take to heal. It is a case of being patient and watching carefully for changes on any level.

If your animal does suffer an aggravation, stop the remedy for about 24 hours and start it again once it has calmed down. If it does not calm down, either wait a bit longer (if the animal is not suffering in any way) or use strong peppermint or coffee as an antidote to the remedy. Remember that an aggravation is a good sign and shows that you have the right remedy. A severe aggravation is unlikely with low potencies, but never risk an aggravation with a very weak or old animal, because it (and you) may not be able to cope.

Giving the remedies

Due to their fragile nature there are some important guidelines to follow when using homoeopathic remedies:

- Do not touch the remedies. Put them straight into the animal's mouth on the container lid or from a plastic spoon.

- If your pet resists taking the remedy (cats often do) you can crush it up in a small amount of milk, butter or anything else your pet relishes, including ice cream!

- Give the remedies away from meals, leaving about half an hour before or after a mealtime.

- If you are using more than one type of remedy at a time, separate them by at least five minutes.

Storing the remedies

The very nature of homoeopathic remedies as an energetic form of medicine makes them fragile and easily damaged. However, if you keep to the following guidelines they should last for quite a few years:

- Store the remedies away from strong smells such as peppermint, camphor, perfume.

- Store in a dark cupboard, keeping away from strong light.

- Store at room temperature.

- Keep the lid on when not in use.

Is homoeopathy compatible with other treatments?

Because homoeopathy works in an holistic way by treating the animal as a whole, it should be given a chance to work on its own before adding other forms of medicine. It complements well some of the more physical treatments and remedies such as conventional veterinary care, chiropractic, herbs and nutrition, but try not to mix it with other energy medicines like acupuncture or healing, as they can interfere with each other.

Homoeopathic alternative to vaccinations

The issue of vaccinations is a controversial one, and there is much debate about whether they may actually be harmful in the long run. Many homoeopaths feel that routine vaccinations, particularly multiple vaccinations, can lead to disease reactions and a breakdown in the immune system.

Homoeopathy offers an alternative to the conventional vaccinations in the form of homoeopathic nosodes (preparations of potentised disease products) which can be used as a preventative, like a vaccine, to protect your pet from specific diseases (including Parvo virus, kennel cough, distemper, feline leukaemia and feline enteritis). Many of these have been tested in trials and found to have a definite effect, and some kennels and shows will accept proof of these as they would proof of conventional vaccination. It is certainly worth considering if you are unsure about medical vaccinations. The use of homoeopathic nosodes is something that should be done by a homoeopathic vet, but it does offer an alternative to the conventional approach (see 'Where to find a homoeopathic vet' at the end of the chapter).

Homoeopathic medicine chest for dogs and cats

The following remedies make up a basic medicine chest for healing simple day-to-day complaints. It is a good idea to buy these in advance so that you have them to hand when you need them.

Aconite For shock, fear and the start of any condition.
Keynote – sudden.

Arnica The first remedy to reach for in cases of bruising, shock, accident or injury, and for stings, sprains and strained muscles. It also helps with post-operative bruising. You can also use arnica ointment, but not on broken skin.
Keynote – 'ouch!'

Belladonna For fevers. If the animal is very hot with dilated pupils, use this fever remedy rather than aconite. It is the main remedy for fevers with redness, heat and dilated pupils. For heat stroke and great thirst.
Keynote – hot.

Calendula cream For minor cuts and grazes, scratches and wounds. Can be used where the skin has broken. Calendula cream is often combined with hypericum for pain relief.

 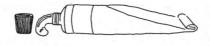

Gelsemium Nervousness is the main use, along with anticipatory fear.
Keynote – trembling.

Hepar sulph For use with abscesses, cat bites, coughs, blocked anal glands or when the glands are up in the neck. Use hepar sulph if you think pus is starting to form, if there is a sudden discharge, or if an area is looking swollen, red or painful. Also for infected wounds.
Keynote – very sore, smelly.

Hypericum Known as the 'homoeopathic painkiller'. Used for injuries where the nerves are affected, post-operative pain, spinal injuries, wounds with shooting pains, puncture wounds and injuries to toes and tails. Can also use hypericum ointment.
Keynote – pain.

Mercury For some diarrhoeas, infections in the mouth, bleeding discharge from the gums, flat teeth that are going to need some dentistry as well to calm the gums down, pus-filled eyes. Also for some discharges, if it is very red and sore.
Keynote – ulcers, smelly.

Nux vomica For digestive upsets, wind, travel sickness, indigestion, some diarrhoeas, vomiting and irritability.
Keynote – irritable, chilly.

Rhus tox For spotty rashes, lameness that is worse just after rest but improves after moving for a while, sprains and strains.
Keynote – spotty.

Sulphur For some diarrhoeas, skin problems, or if you feel an animal is just a bit run down, sulphur is a useful course of treatment.
Keynote – worse for heat.

As you get more experienced you can start adding more remedies to your core stock. When using homoeopathy at home remember to be patient and give the chosen remedy a chance to work before moving on to another one. A lot depends on the condition you are treating, but if you use too many remedies at a time the picture can get muddled and it becomes hard to know what is working and what isn't. In homoeopathy, more is not better – one remedy given at the correct intervals with a large portion of patience is the best way!

'I think homoeopathy for animals is becoming more accepted – or even demanded – now. People are curious. A lot of people expect it to do miracles; it doesn't always, but it can be really satisfying to work with.'
June Third-Carter, VetFMHom

Useful information

Where to buy homoeopathic remedies
Chemists and health-food shops

Weleda UK Ltd
Heanor Road
Ilkeston
Derbyshire DE7 8DR
Tel: 01159 448200
Fax: 01159 448210

Ainsworths Homoeopathic Pharmacy
38 New Cavendish Street
London W1M 7LH
Tel: 0171 935 5330
Fax: 0171 486 4313

Where to find a homoeopathic vet
The British Association of Homoeopathic Veterinary Surgeons
Alternative Veterinary Medicine Centre
Chinham House
Stanford-in-the-Vale
Faringdon
Oxon SN7 8NQ
Tel: 01367 710475
Fax: 01367 718243
They will supply a list of registered homoeopathic vets in the UK.

Further reading
Homoeopathy for Pets, by George MacLeod
A Veterinary Materia Medica and Clinical Repertory, by George MacLeod; C.W. Daniel Company Ltd, 1983
Homoeopathic First Aid Treatment for Pets, by Francis Hunter; Thorsons
Homoeopathy: First Aid for Pets, by Christopher Day; Chinham Publication
The Homoeopathic Treatment of Small Animals, by Christopher Day

CHAPTER THIRTEEN

Osteopathy

At-a-glance guide
What is it? Osteopaths work on an animal's muscles, joints and bones using their hands.
What can it help? Musculo-skeletal problems, injuries, pain relief.
Average cost of treatment? In line with standard veterinary fees, often less.
Can you do it yourself? No. Seek the help of a qualified osteopath who works with animals.
Is it safe? Yes, in the hands of a qualified osteopath.

Osteopathy is a system of diagnosis and treatment, laying its primary emphasis on muscle and joint problems. It is also an holistic treatment, which gives it a greater dimension than just focusing on the body. Osteopathy is a system of whole-body healing.

Osteopathy lends itself well to treating dogs and cats since, like us, they have bones and muscles which can easily get out of alignment or become strained or injured.

Osteopathy and animals
Osteopathy in some form or other has been used for treating animals for a long time – possibly thousands of years – and stems back to the days of the old 'bone setters'. There has always been a tradition where animals have been treated by manual methods, and it was a skill that was passed down through the generations. Modern osteopathy, however, has become scientific and clinical in its approach to both diagnosis and treatment, its educational/training standards and its ever-widening scope.

Osteopathy looks towards the treatment of animals in the same way as it would towards the treatment of humans. An animal's basic structure is the same – they have bones, muscles and joints – and so osteopathy is just as effective with animals as it is with people. In fact, it has been used on animals, particularly dogs and horses, since its inception in the UK in the early part of this century.

What is osteopathy?

Osteopathy is a manipulative treatment working on the body's structure: the skeleton, ligaments, joints, muscles and connective tissues. By adjusting the physical framework and relieving muscle tension, it allows the whole body to work more effectively so that it can begin to heal itself.

Osteopathy is an holistic therapy based on the belief that the body, mind and spirit are connected, a physical problem therefore affecting the harmony of the whole being. In the same way, internal or emotional problems can pop up as structural ones. By relieving the structural problem, other seemingly unrelated ones can disappear too.

How does it work?

Osteopathy is based on the belief that the body has the ability to heal itself and will always try to sort out health problems and bring itself back into balance. However, certain things can get in the way of efficient self-healing – like an accident, poor diet, stress or suppressive drug treatment – and impair the self-healing mechanism. An osteopath will be looking to remove any physical obstacles so that the body's own natural healing mechanism can come into play.

What sort of conditions are commonly treated?

- Arthritis, rheumatism

- Strains

- Joint problems

- Injuries

- Pain

- All kinds of musculo-skeletal problems

Animals can be treated for many of the same things as people – arthritic problems, for example, can be treated quite successfully, and although you cannot cure them, you can make life a lot easier for the animal and take a lot of the pain away. As far as treatment with osteopathy goes, anything that comes under the category of muscle or joint problems usually responds very well.

For specific ailments, see chapter 16.

Treating animals

Animals cannot tell you what is wrong, and so osteopaths have to use their diagnostic skills to try to assess what is going on, based on a knowledge of what the animal should normally be able to do depending on its breed, age, owner's observations and case-history details.

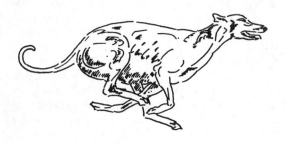

'I treat quite a number of greyhounds. Greyhounds, like all athletes, are highly tuned animals. They tend to have good muscle tone, flexibility and range of movement. Similarly, like all athletes, they must be assessed using sound clinical examination procedures, a knowledge of the kinetics of this athlete in action and a special care for the animal and its sensitivities. Such depth of understanding must be applied not only to the animal, but also to the work of the animal. In this way (taking also the so-very-important case history into account), the animal can effectively be diagnosed and, hence, treated accordingly. It is always very important to insist, however, that the owner procure the written permission of the animal's vet to allow it to be considered for osteopathic intervention.'
Daniel M. Iannarelli, osteopath

What to expect in a treatment

There are a range of techniques that can be used during treatment depending on the osteopath and the nature of the problem, but treatment will usually involve some soft-tissue techniques/massage, gentle articulation/mobilisation of the joints and, if necessary, gentle adjustments to restricted areas.

How many treatments?

Like other forms of natural medicine it is very difficult to know how many treatments your pet might need. All animals will respond to treatment differently, and the number of treatments required also depends on other factors. Generally it takes more than two treatments. Remember that the philosophy behind using natural medicine is that the body has the power to heal itself, given the right conditions. How fast this happens depends on many things: the age of the animal, the extent of its injury, its level of vitality, its immune strength and so on. Because we are so used to fast-acting modern drugs we often forget to be patient with natural medicine.

Case histories

Ben, a ten-year-old tom-cat, suffered from acute tenderness in his hip area. Every time his two-legged flatmate gently touched the low back and hip areas, Ben would jump away in considerable distress. In walking, he seemed to 'limp', particularly on the right side, but there was no evidence of traumatic injury.

Ben had previously been screened by his vet, who could find no obvious injury, nor was there any organic condition present. An X-ray was deemed unnecessary and diagnosis of 'arthritis – due to age' was made. Painkillers were prescribed. Ben was permitted to attend for osteopathic evaluation and treatment.

All the indications of arthritis were present. Passive movements of the hind limb joints all proved restricted and acutely painful. Considering age, examination and presenting symptoms, a diagnosis of osteoarthritis was made, which concurred with the veterinary diagnosis. The treatment involved gentle soft-tissue work (when Ben allowed this) to the muscles of both the low back area and the hips. Gentle articulatory movements were also encouraged to all the joints of the low back and hind limbs. Functional technique/cranial osteopathy was given to round off each treatment. After the second week, Ben seemed to have much less distress in the affected part, and after four weeks there was considerable improvement in movement.

The nature of osteoarthritis being as it is, there is no reversal as such possible. However, a slowing-down of the progress of the condition can be effected, pain lessened (to a degree) and quality of life improved.

'Dwight, a four-year-old greyhound, would limp when running, with head held low. This was unusual for Dwight as, normally (according to his trainer), he tended to walk with his head held high.

'Dwight was first screened by his vet, who could find no obvious injury, nor was there any organic condition present. There was, however, the indication of a mild 'track-leg' condition present, which was affecting the left hind leg and right fore leg. An X-ray was deemed unnecessary and diagnosis of 'left shoulder strain' was made. Painkillers were prescribed. Dwight was permitted to attend for osteopathic evaluation and treatment.

'Dwight showed particular signs of distress in neck/head extension and also in neck/head sidebending to the left. There was acute tenderness on palpation of the C7/D1 vertebral segment, with the tip of the spinous process of C7 deviated to the right. There was no apparent neurological deep-tendon-reflex deficit. After an in-depth osteopathic musculo-skeletal examination, Dwight was assessed as having a restrictive dysfunction at C7/D1, which was probably compressing the left C8 nerve root on its exit from this spinal level – and was thus responsible for the limp.

'Gentle soft-tissue work was given to the muscles of the neck, upper back and shoulder areas. Gentle articulatory movements were also encouraged to all the joints of the neck and shoulders. An adjustment was made to the C7/D1 vertebral level. This regime was carried out twice per week for two weeks. After three treatments, Dwight showed considerable improvement in performance, and no longer had any trouble in keeping his head up. After four treatments, Dwight seemed fully recovered and no further relapses projected.'
Daniel M. Iannarelli, osteopath

Useful information

Where to find an osteopath to treat your pet

Osteopaths are bound by the same rules as other complementary practitioners in that they are not allowed to treat animals unless they are also qualified vets. Most osteopaths who work with animals rely on close co-operation with vets for referrals, and many vets are prepared to refer your pet to a complementary practitioner. If you wish to opt for osteopathy for your pet, the best way to start is by asking your local vet if he can refer you. There is no established association at the moment for osteopaths who work specifically with animals, but the Osteopathic Information Service will give you a list of qualified osteopaths who work with animals.

Osteopathic Information Service (OIS)
PO Box 2074
Reading
Berkshire RG1 4YR
Tel: 01491 875255

Further reading

There are no books specifically on the osteopathic treatment of animals, but if you do wish to find out more about osteopathy generally, the OIS can recommend books on the subject.

CHAPTER FOURTEEN

T-touch Massage

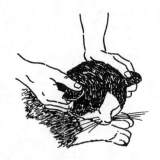

At-a-glance guide
What is it? A way of healing and training animals using touch, gentle massage and exercises.

What can it help? Excellent for behavioural problems and in training situations, musculo–skeletal problems and injuries.

Can you do it yourself? Yes. It is easy to learn and is perfectly safe.

Average cost of treatment? Treatment by a T-touch practitioner will be in keeping with standard veterinary fees, often less. Doing it yourself is free!

T-touch is a way of healing and training animals using touch and body work. It was first developed in Canada by Linda Tellington-Jones, an animal behaviourist, and has recently become very popular in the UK. One of the major benefits of T-touch is that anyone can learn to do it – which makes it a great healing method for treating pets at home.

What is it?

T-touch is a way of working non-habitually with an animal's body to change habitual patterns of behaviour. This makes it a very effective therapy for treating behavioural problems. It is based on Feldenkrais work on humans, which was developed by a man called Dr Moshe. He discovered that by using his body non-habitually – for example, by getting another person to move his body in a non-habitual way, such as circling the leg in a way that he could not do on his own – he was able to create new neural pathways. These new pathways could by-pass damaged neural pathways. Dr Moshe found that by using this method of treatment, he recovered from an old injury that was inhibiting his walking.

Linda Tellington-Jones trained with Dr Moshe and realised the great potential the treatment had for healing animals. She first started using it for horses and then for all animals: dogs and cats, tigers, coyotes, leopards, birds – even whales!

T-touch is a way of working with and training an animal without using fear or force. It is a way of increasing intelligence, because it creates new neural pathways. It can change an animal's posture, and once you change the posture, you change the behaviour. T-touch combines touch, body-work movements and exercises to alter the whole pattern of behaviour of the animal.

How does it work?

It is thought that by opening up new nerve pathways and using non-habitual massage movements, the brain can be activated into changing old habits and negative patterns of behaviour. T-touch bodywork is a way of stimulating cellular intelligence and thereby influencing the whole being of the animal – mind, body and spirit. It can bring about behavioural and personality changes and stimulate the healing of wounds and injuries.

T-touch eases physical tension in the body and opens the neural pathways so that trapped emotions can also be released. Often an animal may become ill as a result of long-held emotions and unpleasant memories.

One of the most important aspects of using T-touch to heal is that it increases the communication between people and their pets. Touch is a powerful therapeutic tool and, used with T-touch, both humans and animals can reach greater levels of understanding with each other. This non-verbal way of communicating with animals through mindful touch is what T-touch is all about. It has been described as allowing you to 'open your heart and speak with your hands'.

Using T-touch with animals

T-touch is a wonderful treatment for animals because it is gentle and effective and strengthens the human–animal bond. It is also harmless and easy to learn.

T-touch involves using repeated, random massage movements over an animal's body. It is different from massage in its intent, which is to wake up the nervous system and make connections between the brain and the body. In a series of small, circular movements, the animal's skin is gently pushed in one and a quarter circles. The circles are made randomly all over the animal's body. This random way of working makes the animal's system wake up and pay attention, inviting movement opportunities the body had not previously thought of or experienced. It is thought that the brain pays attention to something that it is not familiar with, and this allows change to take place on all levels.

T-touch also involves ground–work exercises, depending on the nature of the problem. This may be leading an animal through a specific exercise course which helps them to focus, rebalance and listen to what is being asked of them.

What can be treated?

- All sorts of behavioural problems, such as aggression and excessive barking

- Helpful in training situations and getting rid of bad habits

- Minor injuries and wounds

- Many physical problems, especially musculo–skeletal problems and inhibited mobility

- Pain relief

- Emotional problems, such as fear, nervousness, anxiety

For specific ailments, see chapter 16.

Case histories

'I have worked with aggressive dogs that have become docile, nervous dogs that have become courageous, horses that buck and bite and then stop doing it. T-touch can relieve pain and take away the fear that is trapped within an animal's body, and therefore their behaviour completely changes.'
Sarah Fisher, T-touch practitioner

'I treated a dog, an 11-year-old standard poodle, that had a rear leg ligament injury. The vet said that he thought the dog would eventually have to be put down, because the good leg was going to give way. The dog was compensating by taking his weight off the bad leg and standing on the good leg. He could only lie on one side and he would growl in his sleep. He wasn't able to lift his leg to urinate and had to squat because his knees couldn't support his weight. I worked with him three times, and within one session he was already able to lie more comfortably. Within three sessions he was able to cock both legs! Now his tail is high, his head carriage is amazing, he looks younger than ever and his vet cannot believe it. And that is just from using simple body-work and leading exercises through a labyrinth which helped him to use both sides of his brain and therefore think about both sides of his body.'
Sarah Fisher, T-touch practitioner

Using T-touch on your own pets

The nice thing about T-touch is that it is very user-friendly and you cannot do any harm with it. You can learn the basic movements in half an hour. Regular T-touch massage will keep your pet healthy and prevent small problems becoming major complaints. Another good thing about T-touch is that you can work over an injury site, since it is so gentle. It is also a wonderful way of communicating non-verbally with animals and making them feel loved and cared for.

Consulting a T-touch practitioner

Although T-touch is very easy to learn yourself, there may be times when the problem is too deep-seated or difficult to handle and you may wish to consult someone who is experienced in treating animals in this way. With serious problems, always take your pet to the vet first, and ask them to refer you to a T-touch practitioner if this is the treatment you wish for your pet (see 'Where to find a T-touch practitioner' at the end of the chapter).

Often a T-touch practitioner will work with your pet a few times and then teach you how to continue the treatment at home, along with showing you any relevant ground-work exercises that may be helpful.

Any condition that is serious or that does not show signs of improvement quite quickly should be seen by your vet. Never let a pet suffer.

T-touch is a very safe way of working with an animal and it can help in retraining a dog or cat not to behave in a certain way. By opening up new neural pathways, the animal's whole being can be brought back into a state of health and harmony.

How is it done?

Using the middle three fingers of your hand, gently move your hand over the animal's skin in circular movements, as if you were drawing a clock face. Start at the six o'clock position and draw a complete circle (clockwise), then continue for another quarter circle. Pause, and then move to another part of the body and draw another circle and a quarter. The main emphasis of this body work is that the movements are random and there should be no pattern to them.

It is an easy method to learn and even children can treat their pets in this way. It also teaches both adults and children to communicate with animals and opens up opportunities for greater respect between the two.

T-touch can be done anywhere since it uses little or no equipment, which is why it is becoming such a popular method of healing. It is an effective treatment and can work wonders for pets on many different levels.

How many treatments?

How long treatment takes depends on several factors, including how deep-seated the problems is, the age of the animal and the nature of the problem. Normally you would see results within a day or two. The more severe the problem, the longer it is going to take to heal.

For short-term, acute problems, treatment usually lasts for 15 minutes, two or three times a day. Chronic, long-term problems may need regular daily treatments for several weeks.

Useful information

How to find a T-touch practitioner

T-touch is relatively new to the UK and training courses in T-touch for animals have only recently been set up. To find a practitioner in your area, contact:

Sarah Fisher
South Hill Stables
Radford
Bath BA3 1QQ
Tel: 01761 471182
Fax: 01761 472982

Training in T-touch

Contact Sarah Fisher (details above).
T-touch can also be learned from Linda Tellington-Jones's book and from videos.

Further reading

The Tellington Touch, by Linda Tellington-Jones and Sybil Taylor; Viking Press, 1992

CHAPTER FIFTEEN

Natural Remedies for First-Aid Use

Natural remedies make great first-aid tools, especially when dealing with minor, everyday things like insect bites or cuts and bruises. In more serious situations, such as road traffic accidents or excessive bleeding, natural remedies offer a therapeutic 'stop gap' until your pet can be seen by a vet.

Always seek veterinary help in emergency situations.

It is well worth getting a first-aid kit together before you need it, since you never know when you might have to leap into action. The following first-aid kit contains some of the most useful remedies for first-aid use and can be put together simply and inexpensively. Once you acquire more knowledge about other useful remedies you can build up a larger stock of natural healing aids.

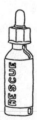

A basic first-aid kit for cats and dogs

1. Bach flower rescue remedy and rescue remedy cream.
   Rescue remedy is the first-aid remedy for all emergency

situations where there is shock, panic, loss of consciousness or trauma. It can help to alleviate stress and calm an animal down enough so that its mind-body healing processes start working without delay.

2. Lavender oil. This helps to soothe and heal burns and repair scar tissue. Lavender reduces inflammation and encourages healing. Useful for treating wounds and abrasions.

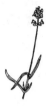

3. Tea tree oil, tea tree cream. Tea tree is effective in killing germs and bacteria. It also has cleansing and antiseptic properties. Can be used neat on burns and insect bites.

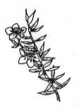

4. Arnica tablets, arnica cream. Arnica is the first remedy to use for any case of shock or injury. It helps to reduce swelling and heal bruised tissue. Emotionally it helps to

calm the nerves after an injury. Do not use arnica cream on broken skin.

5. Calendula cream, calendula tincture. Calendula is used mostly as a topical cream and is a great healing remedy for cuts, burns and bruises. It speeds healing and reduces suppurating.

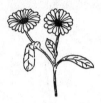

6. Hypericum tablets and tincture. Hypericum is the homoeopathic painkiller. It is particularly good for shooting pain in cases of injury to tails and other extremities. It is also good for cuts and wounds and can be used as a tincture along with calendula to clean wounds. You could also use a combination of calendula and hypericum ointment called hypercal.

7. Witch hazel. Distilled witch hazel used externally helps to reduce inflammation, stop bleeding and ease bruising. Witch hazel is good for cleaning wounds that are still bleeding.

8. Aloe vera gel, aloe vera spray. Aloe vera is a great skin-healer and can be used on cuts, wounds and burns. Aloe vera soothes inflamed skin, protects against infection and speeds the healing process.

9. Comfrey. Used as an ointment on wounds, comfrey is an effective healer once bleeding has stopped. It is especially good for healing broken bones and fractures.

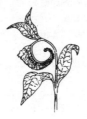

10. Activated charcoal granules/capsules help to delay the absorption of toxins in cases of poisoning. Charcoal also helps with digestive upsets and flatulence.

Accidents

A serious accident, such as when an animal is run over by a car, always requires professional help. Once a vet has been called, natural remedies are the next step. While waiting for the vet to arrive, make sure the animal is moved to a safe place, taking care not to change the position it is lying in to prevent further damage. Keep the animal warm and comfortable and talk to it in a soothing voice. Gentle stroking of uninjured areas, particularly the ears, can be very calming and healing for a distressed animal.

The Bach flower rescue remedy can be given immediately to help calm a distressed animal. Homoeopathic arnica is a useful remedy to alleviate any bruising, along with aconite for shock. All these can be given every ten to fifteen minutes in the early stages following an accident.

Bleeding – excessive/haemorrhage

A small amount of bleeding is quite natural, being nature's way of cleaning out dirt and bacteria, and is not a cause for concern, but excessive bleeding has to be stopped. Severe bleeding can happen if an animal has been in a road traffic accident, got caught on a barbed wire fence or been injured in a vicious dog fight.

Immediately call for help and/or take the animal to your nearest vet. In terms of first aid, the best thing to do in cases of excessive bleeding is to put pressure on the wound using whatever padding you have to hand (this may mean using your clothes) until the bleeding stops. Keep a severely haemorrhaging wound raised higher than the heart and try to keep the animal as calm as possible.

Aromatherapy – Once bleeding has stopped, lavender oil can be used around the wound area, but not on it.

Bach flower remedies – Rescue remedy should be given immediately to calm the animal.

Biochemical tissue salts – Ferr. phos. can be taken internally or used externally on the wound.

Herbs – Goldenseal tincture mixed with water makes a good antiseptic rinse for wounds. A cold compress of witch hazel or rosemary will help to stop bleeding. Aloe vera helps to reduce bleeding and heal wounds and can be used as a spray or as gel applied directly to the wound. Goldenseal and witch hazel can also be used in powder form.

Homoeopathy – Aconite followed by arnica for shock can be given in frequent doses. Calendula lotion can be used locally to help to heal wounds once bleeding has stopped.

Bruising

Aromatherapy – Lavender oil helps to reduce inflammation and encourage healing.

Bach flower remedies – Rescue remedy, especially if the animal has also suffered trauma and stress.

Herbs – Witch hazel can be dabbed on to bruises with cotton-wool to reduce swelling. A cold compress of rosemary tea will help reduce bruising and aloe vera gel applied locally also helps to disperse bruising. Alternatively, apply a slice of raw onion to bruises.

Homoeopathy – Arnica tablets can be taken internally. Arnica ointment can be used topically if the skin is not broken and helps to disperse the bruising. Aconite will help if the animal has suffered stress or trauma as well, and it should be given immediately, followed by arnica.

Burns and scalds

Cats and dogs often burn or scald themselves by jumping up on a hot cooker or chewing through an electric wire. Any serious burn or scald should always be seen by your vet, but minor ones can be effectively treated at home. One of the best things to do immediately is to submerge the burn in cold water, or if that is not possible use a cold water compress or an ice pack on the burn. This will help to cool the skin.

Aromatherapy – Rub lavender oil on the burn. This has soothing and antiseptic properties. Tea tree oil is cleansing and soothing for burns. Geranium helps to heal burns.

Bach flower remedies – Use rescue remedy.

Biochemical tissue salts – Kali. mur. can be given internally or used topically as a lotion. Use calc. sulph. if the burn/scald is suppurating.

Herbs – Aloe vera gel or spray can be applied topically on unbroken skin to accelerate healing. Calendula cream can be used to soothe broken skin.

Homoeopathy – Use arnica for shock and if there is blistering, urtica for continuous stinging pain, cantharis for pain relief. Once blisters have burst, wash the area with diluted calendula tincture two or three times a day.

Honey is very soothing on a burn, and/or use vinegar or a slice of raw potato. Vitamin E can be used directly on burns and scalds.

Cuts and grazes (also see wounds)
Minor cuts and grazes are common in pets and can usually be dealt with adequately at home.

Aromatherapy – Tea tree is the best essential oil for cuts and grazes. It has powerful natural antiseptic and anti-bacterial properties. Lavender oil can also be used. Add a few drops to water to clean the wound.

Bach flower remedies – Use rescue remedy given orally. Rescue remedy cream can be used on the cleaned wound.

Herbs – Aloe vera is a great antiseptic and healer and can be applied topically in gel form or as a spray on a clean wound. You can also use comfrey ointment on a clean wound.

Homoeopathy – Clean the wound with calendula or hypericum tinctures. Give arnica tablets if there is any bruising.

Fractures and broken bones
See musculo-skeletal problems in chapter 16.

Insect bites and stings
Cats and dogs often chase insects and sometimes end up getting stung. Both bites and stings can penetrate the skin and cause swelling, redness and even infection. Always clean the wound before treatment.

Aromatherapy – Lavender oil is soothing and helps to ease stinging and burning sensations. Geranium or tea tree oils help to relieve pain and ease itching.

Bach flower remedies – Give rescue remedy orally. Rescue remedy cream can be used topically on bites and stings.

Biochemical tissue salts – Nat. mur. can be applied externally to the wound in the form of a paste.

Herbs – Marigold ointment can help to reduce swelling. For wasp or bee stings, remove the sting with tweezers, dab some vinegar on the wound and then place a slice of fresh onion over it. A drop of nettle extract (urtica) can ease stings. Aloe vera gel/spray is soothing and cooling and the spray can be used as an insect-repellant.

Homoeopathy – Apis. mel. is soothing for swollen and red stings, such as wasp stings. Use hypericum for horsefly bites. You can use hypericum or hypercal tinctures to clean bite wounds. Calendula ointment can also be applied to bites.

Poisoning

Cats and dogs can be poisoned by all sorts of things, including garden chemicals, slug pellets, household chemicals and medicines. Poisoning can also be the result of an evening's bin-raiding! The most obvious symptoms are vomiting and diarrhoea. Always call your vet if you suspect poisoning, since treatment will vary depending on what the animal has swallowed. It may not always be the best thing to make them sick, so always err on the side of caution and wait for the vet. If possible keep some of the suspected poison (including vomit or diarrhoea) to help identify what it was that they ate.

In terms of first aid, one of the best things to do is to delay the absorption of the poison using activated charcoal granules/capsules. Mix about five heaped teaspoons in a cup of water (or empty out the contents of capsules). Give this mixture to your pet, using a quarter to a full cupful depending on their size. Make sure that you get 'activated' charcoal.

Bach flower remedies – Give rescue remedy. Use crab apple for cleansing, olive for exhausted and sick animals.

Herbs – Milk thistle (silymarin) given afterwards will help to repair any liver damage as a result of the poison. Aloe vera juice is also a good all-round intestinal detoxifier.

Homoeopathy – Give aconite for shock associated with poisoning, nux vomica for poisoning by plants or foods and arsenic for associated pain and restlessness, acute vomiting or diarrhoea. The animal may want to drink little and often.

Shock/trauma/loss of consciousness

Shock and trauma are very common after an accident and an animal will display symptoms of rapid breathing, whitened gums and might also fall unconscious. The first thing to do is to call or visit the vet. In terms of first aid, there is much you can do until professional help arrives.

Aromatherapy – Put a few drops of lavender or peppermint oil on a handkerchief and hold this under your pet's nose. You can also use diluted lavender to massage into their ears – there is a shock point at the tip of the ear which when massaged will help to calm the animal.

Bach flowers – Rescue remedy is a wonderful remedy for all cases of shock. For unconscious animals, lift the flap of their mouth and drop some rescue remedy in, or rub some drops into the fur behind their ears. Star of Bethlehem is also good for trauma or injury.

Biochemical tissue salts – Give nat. sulph. Place the tablets in the mouth of an unconscious animal, where they will quickly dissolve.

Homoeopathy – Aconite is the first remedy to use in all cases of shock, followed by arnica. Place the remedies in the mouth of an unconscious animal, where they will quickly dissolve.

Sprains and strains

See musculo-skeletal problems in chapter 16.

Sunstroke/overheating

The most likely cause of this is when a pet is left in a hot car – they can even fall unconscious. Always park your car in the shade and leave a window open if leaving an animal for any length of time. It only takes a short while for an animal to overheat. Make sure fresh water is also available to them.

Sunstroke and overheating can be fatal, so always call your vet. The next step is to get the animal into the shade and soak them with cool water. If possible use an ice pack around their head to cool the brain and, if they are conscious, see if they will drink some water.

Bach flower remedies – Rescue remedy is the emergency remedy.

Homoeopathy – Use aconite to relieve shock and the early effects of heatstroke. Give belladonna if there is also great thirst.

Wounds

Dogs and cats can be wounded in all sorts of ways, including traffic accidents and fights. Serious wounds, like puncture wounds, always need veterinary attention, but many minor wounds such as scratches, or getting their tail caught in a door, can often be treated at home. Also see cuts and grazes and bleeding.

Aromatherapy – Lavender oil is cleansing and antiseptic and can be used near the wound but not on it. Tea tree oil can be used on wounds and is a powerful antiseptic.

Bach flowers – Use rescue remedy taken orally or used topically as cream. Give star of Bethlehem for trauma and injury.

Biochemical tissue salts – Use ferr. phos. externally and internally, calc. sulph. for suppurating wounds.

Herbs – Aloe vera is a natural antiseptic and can be used to clean the wound (used in spray form). Aloe vera gel rubbed on afterwards reduces bruising and aids healing of damaged tissue. A poultice of slippery elm draws out pus or any foreign bodies from the wound.

Homoeopathy – Arnica helps prevent bruising, stop bleeding and accelerates the healing of damaged tissue. Use ledum for wounds if there is a risk of tetanus, and hypericum for shooting pains often associated with tail injuries. Calendula lotion has remarkable healing properties and can be used directly on wounds. Calendula and hypericum tinctures can be used to clean a wound and can be bought in a combination called hypercal. Goldenseal tincture also makes a good antiseptic rinse.

Vitamins – Vitamin E used topically helps to promote skin healing.

CHAPTER SIXTEEN

Specific Ailments and Treatments

This chapter lists a number of common complaints and conditions which can be helped by natural treatments and remedies. Many of the remedies can be used safely and effectively at home, but if your pet has a serious condition you should always seek veterinary advice.

In the same way as you would assess your own health or a child's health, it is a matter of using your common sense and deciding whether your pet can be effectively treated at home or whether you need to go to the vet. More and more vets are incorporating complementary treatments into their practice, but if your own vet does not practise complementary medicine, ask them to refer you to an holistic vet. Many vets are also happy to refer you to a chiropractor, healer or some other similarly qualified practitioner who treats animals, as long as they are kept up to date with the course of treatment your pet is receiving. Be firm about getting the treatment you want for your pet.

When using natural remedies yourself or seeking professional help for your pet, make sure you understand how the treatments and remedies work and know what you can realistically expect. When used correctly, natural remedies make wonderful healing tools, and the more you can learn about natural medicine, the more you can help your pet to stay healthy and happy. Preventing illness with a good diet and by treating simple things yourself allows you to take a more active and positive role in your pet's health.

Nothing can take the place of preventative medicine, which is why a natural diet and supplement programme is vitally important and will enhance the effects of every other treatment. A complete recovery or a return to optimum health can only happen when your pet is on a good diet, since an inadequate diet may have been the very thing that caused their illness in the first place!

When using the remedies at home, choose one type of treatment at a time. As mentioned earlier, more is not better, and different remedies can interfere with each other. If you choose to use herbs, for example, then pick one or two from the recommended list and let them have a chance to work before trying another herb or another remedy. With homoeopathy, use the remedy that most fits the symptoms and only use another if it does not bring about an improvement. In the same way, it is best to use one treatment type at a time and not book your pet an appointment with a chiropractor, a healer and a homoeopath all in the same week! It is also important to read the chapter on your chosen remedy for information on how to use the remedy and what dose to give. Where relevant, some of the chapters include details of putting together a basic medicine chest for that particular remedy. The more you understand about natural medicine and how to use it, the more responsible you can be for your pet's health.

Remember too that natural remedies work more gently and more slowly than fast-acting modern drugs, so be patient. There may be times when drugs are the only choice, and natural treatments can be used afterwards to support the recovery process.

The following chart is a quick reference guide to the most suitable treatments and remedies for each complaint and condition. Although natural medicine is holistic and will therefore have a positive effect on all disease, be it physical, emotional, mental or spiritual, different treatments can be more effective than others depending on the nature of the problem.

	...ch	...	...pe-y	...s	...ng	...er ces	...practic	...emical Tissue Salts	...a-y	...uncture	...nd Supplements
Behavioural Problems	3	0	2	2	3	3	0	1	2	1	2
Cancer	1	0	2	3	3	1	0	1	1	2	3
Cardiovascular System	1	1	2	2	2	1	1	2	1	2	3
Digestive System	1	1	2	3	3	1	1	2	2	2	3
Ear Problems	0	0	3	3	1	1	0	1	3	1	2
Eye Problems	0	0	3	3	2	1	0	1	1	3	2
Immune System	1	1	3	3	3	2	1	2	2	3	3
Kidney & Urinary	1	1	2	3	2	1	1	2	2	2	3
Muscle & Joint Problems	3	3	2	2	2	1	3	2	2	3	3
Parasites	0	0	2	3	1	1	0	1	2	1	3
Pregnancy	1	2	2	2	1	2	2	1	1	2	3
Respiratory System	1	1	3	3	2	1	1	1	3	3	3
Skin & Coat	1	1	3	3	2	2	1	1	2	2	3
Spaying	3	0	2	2	3	3	0	1	2	2	2
Pain Relief	2	2	2	1	3	1	2	1	2	3	1

Behavioural problems in pets can be caused by a number of things and in many cases there are underlying emotional or mental problems that need to be addressed. Flower remedies and healing are particularly good treatments for behavioural problems, and it is important to read chapters nine and ten to get a fuller understanding of emotional and mental problems in pets and how they can be helped.

Many of the problems displayed by our pets bear a close resemblance to our own behavioural patterns. It is therefore really important to look at the stresses around the home and to remove these in order to bring about a complete change. Pets whose owners are going through a divorce, for example, will display behavioural problems, just like children often do. When treating pets with behavioural problems, very often the owner needs the same remedy.

Many behavioural problems stem back to negative experiences in an animal's early life, and these too can be treated with natural remedies.

Causes of behavioural problems are many and varied and include: poor breeding (viciousness, repetitive habits, nervous-system imbalances), poor nutrition, frequent or multiple vaccinations, inadequate exercise, lack of stimulation and attention, too much attention, excessive attachment to a pet, inappropriate expectations of a pet, and being treated like a human being, not an animal!

Because of its holistic nature, natural medicine has a lot to offer animals with behavioural problems. Suitable treatments include acupuncture, aromatherapy, biochemical tissue salts, diet and supplements, flower remedies, healing, herbs, homoeopathy and T-touch.

Abused animals
See aggression and biting, and nervousness, anxiety and fear.

Aggression and biting
Aggression in the right circumstances is entirely healthy and normal, but inappropriate aggression is not. A dog who bites the postman or a cat who scratches for no reason makes an unpredictable and unsociable pet, and in some cases a dangerous one. Some breeds are more aggressive than others, but on the whole there are underlying

reasons for aggressive behaviour, such as fear, bad breeding, jealousy, past abuse, hyperactivity, stress, allergies, pain and illness. Aggressive behaviour is often a symptom of a deeper underlying emotional or mental problem, and once this is healed, inappropriate aggression will usually disappear.

Diet – A natural preservative-free or allergy diet is an essential first step towards curing behavioural problems which may be caused by an intolerance to particular foods or food additives. Oats have a calming effect and can be made into a porridge. Anti-stress supplements include raw honey, brewer's yeast (or a B-complex vitamin), vitamin C, vitamin E and zinc. You can also give bonemeal or a calcium and magnesium supplement, or a good-quality multi-mineral and vitamin formula (see chapters three and four for details).

Aromatherapy – Touch is an important element in healing disturbed animals and a massage can be very relaxing and calming for them. Sandalwood, ylang ylang and lavender oils can be used for massage or used in a diffuser/burner.

Bach flower remedies – Use chicory for possessiveness, water violet for cats and dogs with a wild ancestry, holly for jealousy and animals quick to become angry and with a tendency to bite, impatiens for irritability, cherry plum for animals who lose control in aggression situations, and beech for intolerance.

Herbs – The most commonly used herbs for soothing and calming are chamomile, skullcap and valerian.

Homoeopathy – Use belladonna for anger and a tendency to bite, nux vomica for irritability and arsenicum for anger and attacks of panic.

Bad habits

Also see spraying (cats), aggression and biting, and nervousness, anxiety and fear.

Bach flower remedies – Chestnut bud is a good remedy for animals with bad habits to break, such as chewing shoes or furniture, or raiding the dustbin. Healing and T-touch may be helpful treatments as well.

Barking/mewing (excessive)
See hyperactivity, bad habits.

Depression
See grief, pining and bereavement.

Eating own faeces or other animals' faeces
See appetite problems, digestive problems, bad habits.

Grief, pining and bereavement
Just like us, animals get attached to places and people and their loss can cause feelings of depression, pain and grief. If a pet's owner dies an animal can become overwhelmed by grief, and many of these animals end up in rescue centres – which further adds to their stress. There are lots of stories about the incredible bonding that can happen between a human being and an animal, and if you have been lucky enough to experience its strength you can appreciate just how emotionally developed animals are. Helping a pet overcome grief takes time, patience and love.

Diet – A good-quality natural diet is very important during stressful times, and it helps to boost an animal's immune system. See stress for helpful supplements. Also see chapters three and four for diet and supplement recommendations.

Aromatherapy – Massage and touch are very therapeutic for depressed or grief-stricken animals. They need more love and attention at this time and will greatly benefit from regular relaxing massages. Use neroli for improved mood, sweet marjoram and lavender to help with sleep, and basil and sweet marjoram for depression.

Bach flower remedies – Star of Bethlehem is good for emotional trauma, past or present, and is especially helpful for animals in rescue centres. Use honeysuckle for grief or homesickness, for an animal that has lost its mate or owner, or when in boarding kennels. Use mustard for depression and mood swings, pine for rejected animals, walnut to help pets adapt to change, crab apple to release negative emotions from the past (e.g. past abuse), and red chestnut for worrying, pining animals waiting for their owner to come home.

Herbs – Use chamomile, skullcap and valerian to calm and reduce stress.

Homoeopathy – Use ignatia for bereavement, pining, grief and homesickness.

Hyperactivity
Hyperactivity in pets includes things like excessive barking or mewing, constantly jumping up and seeking attention, rarely relaxing, becoming easily excited, irritability, biting and scratching, nervousness and anxiety, and being oversexed or difficult to train.

Some cases can be put down to bad breeding, allergies, boredom, stress, insecurity, lack of stimulation, inadequate exercise, lack of routine, excess protein and lack of love and attention. Although some breeds are naturally highly strung, most hyperactivity is rooted in underlying emotional or mental problems, inadequate feeding, stress around the home, and allergies.

Diet – Very often hyperactivity in pets is related to an intolerance to certain foods and food additives. Changing to a natural preservative-free diet is sometimes enough on its own to cure the problem. Oats have a calming effect and can be used as porridge. Specific supplements for hyperactivity include brewer's yeast (or vitamin B complex), vegetable and fish oils, bonemeal (or a calcium and magnesium supplement) and vitamin C. Also see stress and chapters three and four for more details.

Aromatherapy – Massage can be very relaxing for restless, hyperactive pets. Calming oils include lavender, sweet marjoram, basil and chamomile. These can also be used in a diffuser/burner.

Bach flower remedies – Use rock rose for panic attacks, vervain for highly strung, hyperactive animals.

Biochemical tissue salts – Kali. phos. is a good nerve tonic.

Herbs – Use oat straw tincture, skullcap and valerian for calming. Aloe vera and kelp are useful detoxifiers when allergies are suspected.

Homoeopathy – Use scutellaria (skullcap) for highly strung, often destructive pets, belladonna for excitable, aggressive pets.

Moving home

Also see grief, pining and bereavement.

Bach flower remedies – Walnut helps an animal adapt to change. Scleranthus eases travel sickness.

Homoeopathy – Ignatia helps with accepting new surroundings.

Nervousness, anxiety, fear

A nervous, anxious animal is often one that has had a bad experience earlier in its life, such as an accident, abuse, abandonment, frequent change of owner or neglect. Pets can be nervy and highly strung all the time or scared of specific things like thunderstorms, small children, vacuum cleaners and hair dryers. A nervous animal is often unpredictable and may bite or scratch without good reason.

Other causes of nervous behaviour include allergies to foods or chemicals, and physical illness.

Natural remedies can help to calm nervous animals and heal emotional or mental stress that is causing their behavioural problems. With behavioural problems it is always a good idea to evaluate the stress in the home, since your pet may be reacting to its emotional environment. T-touch and healing are effective treatments in addition to those below.

Diet – Behavioural problems are often related to food intolerances, so changing your pet's food to a natural preservative-free or allergy diet is essential. Oats added to the diet have a soothing and calming effect. Certain supplements are helpful in combating stress and can be included in the diet, e.g. vitamins C, E, A and D, B complex, zinc, calcium and magnesium. Use a good-quality multi-vitamin and mineral supplement containing these, or add them individually to the diet. See chapters three and four for details.

Aromatherapy – Massage is relaxing and comforting for anxious pets. Use a combination of the following oils: chamomile, neroli, lavender and sweet marjoram.

Bach flower remedies – Use aspen for anxiety and apprehension, but not specific fears. Use mimulus for specific fears like a fear of thunderstorms, rock rose for terror, extreme fright or panic, rescue remedy for fear and shock, and star of Bethlehem for past traumas not fully recovered from.

Biochemical tissue salts – Kali. phos. is a good nerve tonic.

Herbs – Chamomile, skullcap and valerian are all calming herbs.

Homoeopathy – Use aconite to minimise fear before or after a frightening experience such as fireworks or thunderstorms. Give gelsemium when rigid with fear, phosphorus for fear of sudden noises and argent. nit. for restless, anxious pets.

Oversexed
See hyperactivity.

Spraying (cats)
Usually some kind of stress is at the root of inappropriate spraying, when cats suddenly begin marking the house with urine. Things like a new arrival to the household, moving home or shock can trigger stress-related problems. Natural treatments and remedies work very well for problems like these. Follow the guidelines for stress and nervousness, or use the following specific treatments.

Aromatherapy – Spray areas of the house that your cat sprays with natural repellent aromas like lemon oil, geranium and eucalyptus. They will soon get the message! Dilute a few drops of oil in a base of vodka and water to use as a repellent spray.

Bach flower remedies – Use willow for resentment and anger, chestnut bud for bad habits.

Stress

Stress is something we all seem to suffer from these days, and so do our pets. Many pets do not live a natural life and are fed on what amounts to 'convenience' food for animals. Often dogs get left alone for hours on end in a city flat, and some cats never get outside in their entire lives. All of these things are highly stressful and not a good recipe for mental or emotional health, and eventually animals display behavioural problems as a result.

Our pets also pick up on our stress and mirror our moods. It is therefore a good idea to treat owners and pets with the same remedies! Stress-related diseases are on the increase, and there is a lot you can do to help reduce your own and your pet's stress levels.

Diet – A natural preservative-free diet and supplement programme will enhance your pet's health and help them to cope with stress. Specific supplements for stress include brewer's yeast (or a B complex), vitamins C and E, bonemeal (or calcium and magnesium), zinc, raw honey, royal jelly and oats. See chapters three and four.

Herbs – Ginseng helps the body cope with stress and combines well with royal jelly. Chamomile, oatstraw, skullcap and valerian are all calming.

Massage, healing and T-touch are also excellent for stressed pets.

Also see nervousness, anxiety and fear.

CANCER

Cancerous tissue can grow literally anywhere in or on the body. Sometimes the cancer is obvious, such as a skin tumour, but other times it is not, as is the case with liver cancer. There are many causes of cancer in cats and dogs, including pollution, stress, electrical emissions (televisions, mains supply, etc.), inadequate diet, chemical additives, colourings and preservatives, and unnatural residues in food from intensive farming. Cats and dogs are affected by pollution in the environment, food and water just as we are, and this damages their immune system. If the immune system is damaged, the body's natural ability to fight cancerous cells is impaired.

Natural remedies and treatments can help to alleviate symptoms and boost the immune system to fight against cancer. (Also see immune system.) The emphasis is always on prevention, so that your pet is not exposed to excess pollutants in their food, water or environment in the first place. If an animal can be kept in peak health, its immune system will remain strong and it will be more resistant to cancer-causing agents. An unnatural diet is a major factor in cancer, whereas a natural diet boosts the animal's own powers of self-healing and resistance to disease.

Suitable treatments include acupuncture, aromatherapy, diet and supplements, flower essences, healing, herbs and homoeopathy.

Before treating your pet at home, always read the relevant chapters on the treatments and remedies you are planning to use for information on dosage and how each of the treatments works. In the case of serious disease you may need to combine conventional drugs with natural remedies.

Diet – A natural preservative-free diet is the most important factor in the prevention and treatment of cancer. Use organic foods where possible, especially if your pet already has cancer, to make sure the diet is as pollutant-free as possible. Use filtered or bottled mineral water, not tap water. Helpful foods in the diet include dried apricots, carrots, broccoli, potatoes, watercress, beetroot, cabbage, turnip and garlic. Raw sweetbreads (thymus) and liver are also 'positive' foods (see chapter four). Apple cider vinegar added to food or water helps to keep the internal acid/alkaline balance right, which is important in preventing and arresting the spread of cancer. Also give B-complex vitamins, high doses of vitamin C (double the normal dose), vitamin A (1,000–3,000iu), vitamin E (200–600iu), royal jelly, kelp and alfalfa.

Oats are strengthening. In addition, give fish oils, evening primrose oil and vegetable oils, along with a good-quality multi-mineral and vitamin complex or added kelp and alfalfa for nutrients.

Aromatherapy – Ylang ylang and rosemary are revitalising and can be used in a diffuser or massaged into your pet's skin.

Herbs – Mistletoe has anti-tumour properties. Immune-strengthening herbs include garlic, aloe vera and echinacea. Milk thistle strengthens and repairs the liver. Oat tincture is strengthening. Aloe vera and liquid chlorophyll help to detoxify the system.

Homoeopathy – Use hydrastis in early cases of cancer. Arsen. alb. relieves pain. Use thuja for warty tumours. Viscum. alb. is beneficial in most cases of cancer.

The cardiovascular system includes the heart and blood and the circulatory system. Heart and circulation problems are relatively common in older pets and include things like a weak heart muscle, high blood pressure, thickening of the heart muscle, heart failure, an irregular pulse and anaemia.

Some of the commonest causes of heart problems are a high-stress lifestyle, hereditary factors, poor nutrition, pollution and toxic chemicals in food and water.

Signs to look out for if you suspect your pet has heart trouble are laboured breathing, a persistent dry cough, coughing after exercise or during the night, fluid retention in the legs and abdomen and extreme nervousness. There may also be a bluish look to the tongue and gums.

Any heart or circulation problems should always be checked out by your vet, since poor circulation can ultimately affect other organs like the liver and kidneys.

Heart disease can be prevented by giving your pet a healthy, low-stress lifestyle, nutritious food and regular exercise. Natural treatments and remedies can help treat heart and circulation problems and work well as a preventative measure.

Suitable treatments include acupuncture, aromatherapy, bio-chemical tissue salts, chiropractic, diet and food supplements, flower essences, healing, herbs, homoeopathy and T-touch. Before treating your pet at home read the relevant chapters for information on treatment, remedies, dosage, suppliers, etc.

Heart and circulation problems

Diet – Pets fed on natural diets rarely get heart disease. Processed foods and inadequate diet are two of the biggest contributory factors, so change your pet's diet to one that is natural and preservative-free. Sugar (including honey) and salt should be entirely omitted. The diet needs to be low on meat protein, so use tofu and eggs as alternative protein sources. Add raw vegetables and whole cooked grains. Watercress is a good circulation tonic. Use only filtered or bottled water. Apple cider vinegar adds potassium. For overweight dogs, see weight problems/obesity. Useful supplements include royal jelly, magnesium, calcium, B complex, vitamin C, vitamin E (not for very weak hearts until stabilised), cod liver oil (or vitamins A and D), magnesium and calcium, evening primrose oil, lecithin and digestive enzymes. Seaweed is also an excellent supplement for keeping the blood and circulation healthy – every mineral normally found in healthy blood is found in seaweed (see chapters three and four for details).

Exercise – Moderate regular exercise is good for the heart and circulation.

Aromatherapy – Massage with lavender, clary sage, ylang ylang, mint and ginger.

Bach flower remedies – Use oak for strengthening very weak animals, impatiens for nervousness, and hornbeam for weak, fatigued animals.

Biochemical tissue salts – Use kali. phos. if problem is due to nervous excitement. Calc. flour. restores strength to the heart muscle.

Herbs – Use alfalfa for added nutrients. Hawthorn berry tincture is a heart muscle repairer and general heart tonic. Dandelion, parsley and watercress are mildly diuretic. Use ginger to stimulate circulation, and skullcap to calm. Garlic lowers blood pressure and cholesterol. Kelp lowers high blood pressure. Aloe vera is rich in minerals and chlorophyll.

Homoeopathy – Crataegus (hawthorn berries) is the main remedy for heart problems with breathing difficulty, irregular/weak pulse, high blood pressure, fluid retention, weak heart, irritability and nervousness.

Anaemia

Anaemia is a lack of red blood corpuscles in the blood. It is the red blood corpuscles which carry oxygen round the body to the organs and tissues, and they are therefore vital to life. Causes of anaemia include blood loss from wounds, parasites (fleas and worms), underproduction of red blood corpuscles, internal bleeding and poisons, e.g. warfarin (rat poison), heavy-metal poisons like lead. Underproduction of red blood corpuscles can be caused by iron deficiency, inadequate diet, viruses and kidney disease.

Signs and symptoms of anaemia include sluggishness, lack of energy and vitality, pale gums and pale membranes around the inner rim of the eyelid, weight loss, lack of appetite and depression. Always take your pet to your vet for a diagnosis in case there is a serious underlying problem.

Diet – Change to a natural preservative-free diet as recommended in chapter three. Increase the amount of iron-rich foods such as red meat, liver, eggs, lentils, green leaf vegetables, spinach, watercress, blackstrap molasses and red foods – beetroot, black grapes, red pepper and apricots. Prunes, figs and raisins are also 'positive' foods for anaemia. Digestive enzymes will help with the absorption of nutrients. Kelp and liquid chlorophyll add valuable extra nutrients. When it comes to supplements, use a good-quality multi-vitamin and mineral complex which includes vitamin C, B complex, vitamin B12, folic acid (or give brewer's yeast for the B group of vitamins), copper, calcium and magnesium. Vitamin C and copper help the absorption of iron (see chapter four).

Aromatherapy – Wild marjoram will help to invigorate tired, exhausted animals.

Bach flower remedies – Use olive for exhaustion or an ill animal, hornbeam to strengthen.

Biochemical tissue salts – Use ferr. phos. and calc. phos.

Herbs – Use alfalfa, dandelion, nettle and parsley. Nettle and parsley in particular supply plenty of iron and vitamin C.

Homoeopathy – Use ferrum. met. if inadequate nutrition is a factor, phosphorus for persistent bleeding leading to anaemia, china after blood loss leading to weakness, nux vomica after blood loss with irritability and silicea for underlying constitutional factors.

The digestive system starts in the mouth and ends at the anus and includes the stomach, intestines, liver, kidneys and pancreas. This section covers many of the more common problems relating to the whole digestive process, including dental disease; weight problems; colic; colitis; liver, kidney and pancreatic disease; constipation and diarrhoea; malabsorption; bad breath; flatulence; allergies and travel sickness. The single most important treatment for digestive problems is a good diet; it is therefore essential to read chapters three and four if treating any of the following complaints.

Suitable treatments include acupuncture, aromatherapy, biochemical tissue salts, diet, food supplements, flower essences, healing, herbs and homoeopathy. Before treating your pet at home, read the relevant chapters for information on treatment, remedies, dosage, suppliers, etc.

Allergies

Allergies or food sensitivities are on the increase both in humans and in pets, and many people would say it is because our food and environment are becoming increasingly polluted and our lifestyles more stressed and unhealthy.

An allergic reaction is an adverse response by the immune system to something that is normally harmless to the body, such as wheat, beef or plant pollen. Reactions can range from sneezing and watery eyes to diarrhoea and skin rashes. Contributing factors are a poorly functioning digestive system, an overburdened or weakened immune system or weakened liver function due to excess toxins and stress.

The most common trigger foods are milk, beef, pork, chicken, wheat gluten, soya, food additives, grasses, pollens, moulds, house dust, house dust mites, fleas, household chemicals and washing powder. Reactions can be many and varied, including skin problems, itching, scratching, inflamed ears, digestive upsets, diarrhoea, constipation, urinary tract infections, vomiting, hair loss, rashes, hyperactivity and other behavioural disturbances.

There is a lot that can be done with natural treatments, although it can take time and effort. (Also see skin and coat problems, fleas, immune system and other relevant ailments.)

Diet – About a third of allergies are thought to be caused by food, therefore fasting and a change of diet is the best way to start (see

163

chapter three). By reducing your pet's diet to a few foods (preferably organic) and then gradually reintroducing more foods, the 'triggers' can usually be spotted and subsequently avoided. Commercially made pet food contains many potential allergens such as chemicals, colourings, preservatives, flavourings, pesticides and fertiliser residues. Drinking water needs to be filtered, or use bottled spring water. As supplements, give digestive enzymes, acidophilus and a good-quality multi-mineral and vitamin complex. Also give additional vitamin C (500–5,000mg daily), and a non-yeast source of vitamin B complex (see chapter four).

Environment – Eliminate any possible environment triggers such as commercial flea collars, flea powder, insecticides, room deodorisers, strong chemical cleaners and tobacco smoke.

Bach flower remedies – Use rescue remedy for sudden, uncomfortable reactions, crab apple for cleansing.

Herbs – Echinacea, garlic and goldenseal help build the immune system. Use aloe vera and liquid chlorophyll for detoxification and healing the gut. Chamomile will help soothe an allergic response. Use milk thistle (silymarin) and dandelion to support the liver.

Also see specific symptoms, e.g. runny nose, diarrhoea, skin rashes.

Appetite problems

Appetite problems include lack or appetite, excessive appetite or depraved appetite (e.g. eating own faeces).

LOSS OF APPETITE

This is often a sign of illness and animals will naturally fast when they are feeling unwell. During a fast, energy is directed away from digestion towards healing. Once they begin to feel better they will soon want to eat again. If the problem does not resolve itself fairly quickly, take your pet to the vet for a thorough examination. Loss of appetite can be a sign of a range of illnesses from worms or fur balls to diabetes and pancreatic disease.

Dogs usually have good appetites, but cats can develop finicky eating to the extent that they will only eat a few select foods. Try not to let this happen. It is always best to keep a wide range of foods in your pet's diet and if they don't eat it at one meal, take the food away and dish it up at the next. A healthy cat will eventually eat when it gets hungry enough! Most pets who are finicky eaters are given snacks between meals, or their dish is left around with food in it between meals. This encourages fussy eaters! Cats are also prone to becoming anorexic, especially if they have had a trauma, an operation or just feel that their life is over and stop eating. Bach flower remedies can help when emotional reasons lie behind appetite loss. To encourage eating try 'lacing' their food with tempting flavours and ingredients until they get back to normal eating again.

Diet – Change to a natural preservative-free diet which can be 'laced' with tasty bites to encourage eating. Feed small meals at a time and take the food away if your pet does not eat it within half an hour. As a supplement, give a good-quality multi-mineral and vitamin complex. Add extra zinc to make a daily allowance of 5–20mg. Zinc deficiency is strongly indicated in anorexia and a lack of taste or smell which may be the underlying cause of poor appetite.

Bach flower remedies – Loss of appetite is often linked to emotional factors – refer to chapter nine for appropriate remedies.

Herbs – Herbs which stimulate appetite include peppermint, watercress and chamomile.

Homoeopathy – Use arsen. alb. for pets who seem interested in eating but then change their mind. Give carbo. veg. for loss of appetite due to digestive upsets.

See also underweight.

EXCESSIVE OR DEPRAVED APPETITE

An excessive or depraved appetite is usually a sign that the animal is not getting a good-quality nutritious diet or that it is not absorbing nutrients properly because its digestion is at fault. Sometimes pets will eat their own or other animals' faeces in an attempt to get nutrients. Other causes of excessive or depraved appetite include intestinal worms, heart disease and pancreatic or liver disease.

Diet – This is the most important thing to address. First change their diet to a natural preservative-free diet, since allergy or incorrect diet may be the underlying cause. If malabsorption is the problem, the digestive process can be helped by adding digestive enzymes and stomach acid supplements to their food. Acidophilus helps to get the right intestinal environment for optimum absorption of nutrients. A toxic intestinal system can also impede nutrient absorption, therefore psyllium husks added to food will help to clean out the bowel and remove toxins.

Herbs – Aloe vera juice is rich in easily absorbed nutrients and can be added to food. Also use alfalfa tablets, which can be crushed into food, or liquid chlorophyll.

Homoeopathy – Use calc. carb. for depraved appetite in fat animals, calc. phos. for thin animals.

Also see weight problems and parasites.

Bad breath

The most common cause of bad breath is gum disease, so it is worth checking this out first (see also teeth and gums). Other causes of bad breath include digestive problems, liver and kidney problems or worms (see also parasites).

Colic

Colic is a gripping spasmodic pain in the animal's abdomen which can either come in intervals or happen so regularly that it seems like one continuous spasm. Symptoms of colic include obvious discomfort, gurgling noises in the stomach, flatulence, panting, distress and whining or mewing with pain. The most common causes are inadequate diet, impaired digestion and allergies.

Diet – Colic is a sign that the digestive system is not working properly or that the diet is at fault. A change of diet to a natural preservative-free diet is essential. You may also need to add digestive enzymes to your pet's food in the initial stages of healing and use acidophilus powder (friendly gut bacteria). Alfalfa helps with the assimilation of nutrients. Watercress aids digestion. (See also colitis, flatulence and parasites.) Follow the dietary guidelines in chapters three and four.

Aromatherapy – Chamomile, peppermint and caraway oils can be massaged into the abdomen.

Bach flower remedies – Use crab apple for cleansing.

Biochemical tissue salts – Use mag. phos. with cramps, combination E for colic pains, indigestion and flatulence.

Herbs – Aloe vera has a soothing effect on the digestive system. Also use slippery elm, goldenseal, ginger, chamomile and peppermint. Parsley and fenugreek are digestive tonics. Liquorice is anti-inflammatory and soothing.

Homoeopathy – Use nux vomica for chronic cases, colocynthis for acute cases where the pain comes in waves.

Colitis

Colitis is an inflammation of the colon (large intestine) and can be acute (short-term) or chronic (long-term). Signs that your pet is suffering from colitis include diarrhoea or constipation, frequent bowel movements, straining, blood and/or mucus in the stools, abdominal pain and weight loss. There is a wide range of causes of colitis, but a few of the more common ones are allergies, stress, parasites and inadequate diet.

Diet – Diet is the most important factor in treating digestive problems and although colitis may be difficult to cure completely, it can be kept well under control with dietary measures. A high-fibre diet is very important for both dogs and cats, and one of the main ingredients of the diet should be cooked brown rice. Other helpful foods include live yoghurt, oats, carrots, apples and cabbage. If your pet has colitis you should also suspect allergies, especially to wheat gluten (see chapter three). Add acidophilus (friendly gut bacteria) powder or capsules to food (⅛–½ teaspoon per day). Capsules can be opened and sprinkled on to food. Use vegetable and fish oils. Pets with colitis may not be absorbing food completely and will need additional nutrients until they heal, so add a good-quality multi-mineral and vitamin supplement daily. Alfalfa and kelp add valuable nutrients (see chapters three and four).

Biochemical tissue salts – Use mag. phos. for cramping pains.

Herbs – Garlic helps to keep the right internal environment for the friendly gut flora and has an anti-spasmodic effect in the colon. Liquorice is also soothing and has an anti-inflammatory effect on the gut. Fenugreek, peppermint, comfrey, aloe vera and slippery elm can bring relief and ease discomfort.

Constipation

Constipation can be caused by a number of things, although incorrect diet is usually at the root of the problem. Not enough fibre in the diet is the commonest cause, but sometimes animals who have been eating bones get short-term problems, and fur balls can cause constipation in cats (cats need regular grooming to avoid this problem). Lack of exercise and worm infestation are also considerations. If a change of diet does not sort the problem out, consult your vet, since more serious causes of constipation include cancer or a constricted bowel.

Symptoms of constipation in your pet include straining to have a bowel movement, going for long periods between bowel movements (dogs and cats should have at least one or two a day), and hard, impacted faeces.

Long-term constipation can lead to more serious problems, such as bowel cancer, bad breath, skin problems and obesity. If animals are not eliminating properly, they get a build-up of toxic waste in the body which effectively poisons them and causes further health problems.

Diet – Change to a natural preservative-free diet. Make sure they get a good balance of protein, whole grains and vegetables. Include lots of fibre in your pet's meal, such as brown rice, oats, raw grated vegetables (carrots, parsnips, beetroot, cabbage), prunes, figs (fresh or dried) and grated apple. Oils, such as olive oil or sunflower oil (½–3 teaspoons daily), help to lubricate the bowel and alleviate constipation. Make sure your pet has access to fresh drinking water at all times. As supplements, use acidophilus daily, digestive enzymes with meals and linseeds (soaked overnight and added to food). Also use a good-quality multi-mineral and vitamin complex and additional vitamin C (500–5,000mg), which is a great cleanser.

Exercise – Sluggish animals can get constipated, so make sure they get adequate exercise for their breed and age.

Aromatherapy – Massage the lower abdomen with olive oil and a few drops of sage or rosemary.

Bach flower remedies – Use crab apple for cleansing. Stress, anxiety and emotional upsets can all cause constipation – refer to chapter nine for an appropriate remedy.

Biochemical tissue salts – Use nat. mur. for constipation alternating with diarrhoea.

Herbs – Aloe vera is cleansing and soothing. Psyllium husks add fibre to the bowel and help to clear out toxic waste (⅛–1 teaspoon per day in food). If the constipation has been going on for a while, try one or more of the laxative herbs such as rhubarb, senna pods or cascara sagrada.

Homoeopathy – Nux vomica is the basic constipation remedy. Use sulphur if there is also a skin disorder. Use carbo. veg. for simple constipation with gas, or calc. carb. if the constipation is associated with hard, chalky stools and eating bones.

Diabetes

Diabetes is a disease of the pancreas which affects the body's ability to control its blood sugar levels. It is the pancreas's job to produce a hormone called insulin which keeps blood sugar levels balanced, but if this is not happening, glucose cannot be transferred from the blood for use in the cells. A diabetic animal will naturally drink more water to flush the excess sugar out of its system, but this also causes essential minerals and vitamins to be washed out, so although the animal may be eating plenty of food, it is also starving.

The main symptom of diabetes is excess thirst and frequent urination. Other signs and symptoms include lethargy, sugar in the urine and weight loss despite a good appetite. Causes of diabetes include obesity, unhealthy diet (some commercial pet foods are high in sugar and preservatives), cortizone treatment, stress and shock.

Diabetes is a very serious disease and should always be treated by a vet. Your pet may need to have insulin injections for the rest of its life. Other health problems associated with diabetes include cataracts, liver and kidney disease, increased infections and heart disease.

Natural medicine and conventional medicine work well together to treat diabetes and there is much that can be done, especially with diet, to help control blood sugar levels and reduce or even remove the need for long-term use of insulin. Always let your vet know what you are doing, since insulin levels may need to be reduced in line with dietary changes. Never experiment with treating diabetes on your own without veterinary supervision – you could kill your pet.

Diet – A natural preservative-free diet is essential, along with additional supplements. The key word with diabetes is routine, so make sure that your pet's meals are always at the same time every day. Several small meals a day rather than one big one will also help with blood sugar control. Make sure the diet is based on whole grains (rice, millet, oats, cornmeal), lean meats (chicken, turkey), eggs, fish, raw vegetables (carrots, green beans, alfalfa, Brussels sprouts, parsley, onions, garlic) and some fruit (given separately), plus supplements. Above all, avoid commercially prepared dog foods, especially the semi-moist ones, as these contain high amounts of sugar and preservatives. The only way to be sure your pet's food is free of sugars and preservatives is to make it yourself from scratch.

Supplement the diet with a good-quality multi-mineral and vitamin complex and brewer's yeast or a yeast-free B complex. Trace minerals are important for blood sugar control, especially chromium (as glucose tolerance factor), zinc and manganese – make sure these are contained in your multi-mineral supplement or add them according to body weight. Brewer's yeast contains manganese and chromium, and wheat germ contains chromium. Giving vitamin E (25–200iu daily) reduces the need for insulin. Also give vitamin C (500–5,000mg), and pancreatic or digestives enzymes (see chapters three and four).

Exercise – Regular exercise is an important factor with diabetes. A diabetic pet needs a strict routine, so try to exercise them at the same times every day.

Aromatherapy – Eucalyptus, juniper and lemon can be used for massage.

Bach flower remedies – Hornbeam and olive can help to build up a weakened animal.

Herbs – Goldenseal helps with lowering blood sugar. Garlic and liquid chlorophyll are also blood sugar balancers. Also use dandelion and parsley.

Homoeopathy – The main remedy for diabetes is syzygium.

Diarrhoea

Diarrhoea is not always a sign of illness. It has lots of causes, many of which are just the body's natural way of getting rid of irritants such as food allergies, bacterial or viral infections, worms and toxins. In these cases, the diarrhoea usually stops once the toxins have been evacuated, and as long as there are no other signs of illness it is best to leave your pet to it. Other factors, such as a change of diet or stress, can also bring on mild diarrhoea. Some animals will naturally seek out plants that will give them diarrhoea as a way of detoxifying their system. A short-term attack of diarrhoea is not usually a worrying sign, but long-term diarrhoea is and an animal can get very dehydrated and lose essential nutrients. If there is blood or mucus in the stools, tarry, black-coloured stools or if the diarrhoea is accompanied by other symptoms of illness, take your pet to the vet. Puppies and kittens should always be taken to the vet at the first sign of diarrhoea since they can dehydrate very quickly and can even die without swift treatment.

Symptoms of diarrhoea are loose, watery stools, and there may also be belching and wind. Sometimes blood, mucus or undigested food is present in the stools and the animal may also vomit.

Mild, short-term diarrhoea can be treated at home, but long-term, serious problems should always be seen by your vet. If the diarrhoea continues for more than two or three days, a visit to the vet is essential. *Diet* – At the onset of diarrhoea, the most important treatment is a day's fasting. Make sure your pet has plenty to drink. Vegetable broths (the strained liquid only), brown rice water, barley water, apple cider vinegar water or honey water can all be given during the fast to support basic nutritional needs, while at the same time letting nature take its course. When giving food again, change to a natural preservative-free diet, since your pet may be sensitive to preservatives, colourings and other additives in commercially prepared foods. Give acidophilus daily, along with a good-quality multi-vitamin and mineral complex once the fast has finished. If the diarrhoea persists then give activated charcoal tablets (see chapters three and four).

Aromatherapy – Chamomile, geranium and sandalwood can be added to olive oil and massaged into the abdomen to soothe the digestive tract.

Bach flower remedies – Use crab apple for cleansing.

Biochemical tissue salts – Use nat. mur. for thin, watery diarrhoea, or diarrhoea which alternates with constipation. Use nat. phos. for foul-smelling, green stools, and combination S for stomach upsets.

Herbs – Garlic helps to fight infections. Slippery elm, as a syrup, powder or tea, is soothing and nourishing. Aloe vera juice is soothing and adds nutrients. Parsley and fenugreek are digestive tonics.

Homoeopathy – Use arsen. alb. for watery stools, arsenic for vomiting and diarrhoea, merc. cor. for frequent diarrhoea with straining but no vomiting.

Flatulence

Also see stomach problems, constipation, diarrhoea.

Flatulence is caused by a build-up of gas in the stomach or intestines and can be accompanied by bloating, abdominal pain, belching and wind. Undigested food fermenting in the stomach is the commonest cause of excessive gas and it usually responds well to a natural preservative-free diet of the type outlined in chapter three. In most cases a change of diet will be enough to sort out the problem. Food sensitivities can also cause flatulence. Use acidophilus powder, digestive enzymes and stomach acid to assist optimum digestion. Activated charcoal granules/tablets can also help.

Aromatherapy – Peppermint can be massaged around the abdomen.

Biochemical tissue salts – Use mag. phos. or combination E for flatulence and indigestion.

Herbs – Aniseed, caraway, peppermint and fennel all help to reduce flatulence.

Homoeopathy – Use carbo. veg. for most cases, nux vomica when accompanied by diarrhoea and digestive upset.

Fur balls (cats)

Cats groom themselves much more often than dogs and are therefore more prone to swallowing their own hair, which gathers in the stomach forming hair balls. This is usually vomited up as knotted clumps of hair or passed out of their system in the faeces, especially if the cat's diet has adequate fibre and oils in it. The problem can become serious if their digestive system is weak or their nutrition inadequate, because then the hair balls can get stuck and act like a cork in their system – giving rise to diarrhoea followed by constipation, recurrent vomiting, lack of appetite, a build-up of toxins and, eventually, infection. You will know when your cat has a problem with fur balls when it vomits without bringing anything up, vomits foam without hair, or retches in an unsuccessful attempt to bring something up.

Prevention is always better than cure. Regular grooming of cats, especially while they are moulting in the spring and autumn, reduces the amount of hair they might swallow.

Diet – Make sure their diet has plenty of fibre, fats and oils in it to help the hair pass through the digestive system (see chapters three and four).

Herbs – Psyllium husks add fibre to the diet and help remove toxins from the bowel. Aloe vera juice also helps to prevent constipation and has a healing and soothing action on the intestines.

Homoeopathy – Nux vomica is the primary remedy for fur balls and will help the animal to vomit or pass it through the bowel.

Liver disease

The liver has many varied functions, including being a major player in the digestive process and in the elimination of toxins. Any liver condition, therefore, can have serious consequences and should always be seen by your vet first. However, there is a lot you can do with natural remedies that will support liver function and help it to regain health.

Signs of liver problems include vomiting, weight loss, odd-coloured stools, diarrhoea, increased thirst, swollen abdomen and lethargy.

Diet – Diet is the most important treatment for liver conditions, since a well-balanced natural diet can reduce the liver's digestive and detoxification workload. Chemical additives, artificial preservatives and colouring, medical drugs, heavy metals, and so on, all have to be processed by the liver; therefore the less of these your pet takes in, the better it is for its liver.

Change to a preservative-free natural diet, avoiding red meats and milk. The diet should be low in fats and made up of lean meats, eggs, cooked whole grains, and include raw vegetables (carrots and beetroot). Give a good-quality multi-vitamin and mineral supplement daily, along with additional vitamin C (500–2,000mg daily) and lecithin granules (one to three teaspoons added to meals). Use only filtered or spring water, not tap water. Use acidophilus powder and digestive enzymes. Garlic and apple cider vinegar are also helpful additions to the diet (see chapters three and four).

Aromatherapy – Rosemary and mint can be massaged around the liver area.

Bach flower remedies – Crab apple is cleansing. Use hornbeam for a sickly animal, impatiens for an irritable, touchy animal.

Herbs – Dandelion and milk thistle are gentle and supportive for the liver. Swedish bitters are a liver tonic and can be found in health-food shops – mix it with some honey to make it palatable! Do not use herbal tinctures preserved in alcohol in cases of liver disease.

Homoeopathy – Use nux vomica for liver conditions and digestive upsets, chelidonium majus for jaundice and liver complaints.

Pancreas problems
Also see diabetes.

In terms of digestion the pancreas produces digestive enzymes which helps to digest food. If it does not produce enough enzymes, you get a situation where your pet is literally 'starving in the midst of plenty' because it cannot digest and absorb nutrients properly. Symptoms include weight loss, diarrhoea and lethargy. Most cases can be helped with a good-quality natural diet and digestive enzyme supplements. (See also underweight.) The pancreas also has the job of keeping blood sugar levels stable. (See also diabetes.)

Stomach problems (gastritis)
Also see vomiting.

Cats and dogs get upset stomachs just like us, and in most cases it is not serious. The sort of things that cause upset are indigestion, eating food that has gone off (e.g. a result of dustbin-raiding), swallowing hair, swallowing small, hard objects, eating poisons (e.g. weed-killer), travel sickness and allergies. Other more serious causes can be liver, kidney or pancreatic disease or worms. Gastritis is an inflammation of the stomach.

Symptoms include being sick, along with one or more of the following: diarrhoea, abdominal pain, excessive gas, bloating, loss of appetite and listlessness. There may be fever in some cases.

Diet – The most important thing is to change your pet's diet to a preservative-free diet. Food allergy is often the cause of stomach upsets, especially an allergy to cow's milk and wheat gluten. Your pet may have a weak intestinal system and be prone to upsets, in which case a natural, homemade diet which contains fewer toxins will help to ease and strengthen their digestive system. Fasting for the first day or two of stomach upsets really helps to clear out toxins. Follow the guidelines for fasting in chapter three.

Once your pet is eating again, digestive enzymes should be added to meals to aid digestion, along with a good-quality mineral and vitamin supplement, brewer's yeast and acidophilus powder (see chapter four).

Bach flower remedies – Use crab apple for cleansing, agrimony for indigestion caused by stress, hornbeam to help strengthen a sickly animal.

Biochemical tissue salts – Use combination S for stomach upsets.

Herbs – Chamomile and peppermint tea are soothing for the stomach and help indigestion. Aloe vera helps to cleanse and soothe digestive problems. Parsley, dandelion and slippery elm are good digestive healers; alfalfa, aloe vera and slippery elm offer extra nutrients as well.

Homoeopathy – Nux vomica is the classic remedy for digestive problems. Use arsen. alb. with accompanying diarrhoea, phosphorus where vomiting follows eating.

Teeth and gums

Pets get tooth decay and gum disease just like us. However, the better their diet, the less likelihood there is of serious dental problems developing. If you give them sugary treats, then stop it now! Animals do not need them and many are just as happy to munch on raw carrots or nutritious homemade biscuits (see chapter three).

It is a good idea to check your pet's teeth and mouth regularly for early signs of dental decay and gum disease. A build-up of tartar can lead to inflamed gums, infections and tooth decay. Some of the most obvious symptoms are bad breath, inflamed or swollen gums (gingivitis), bleeding gums, excessive salivation, loose teeth, build-up of tartar, pain when eating and loss of appetite.

Serious dental problems should always be treated by a vet, but there is a lot you can also do with natural remedies and a corrective diet at home. Prevention is the key word with dental problems.

Diet – Diet is the single most important factor in avoiding dental problems and keeping teeth and gums healthy. Raw food, which is hard and crunchy, exercises teeth and jaws and helps to remove tartar. Cats that roam freely outside will naturally hunt for small animals and birds, and those that cannot get out can be given chicken bones to chew on. (Never give chicken bones to dogs.) Dogs love raw marrowbones and these can be given on a regular basis. Dried food does not clean teeth and pets that are given a dried-food diet often have the worst teeth. One of the best foods to give your pet regularly is raw meat, especially the tougher cuts like stewing steak or chuck steak, because it not only exercises the jaw but contains connective tissue which acts like dental floss! Raw meat can also help to scrape away some of the tartar.

A multi-mineral and vitamin supplement will build up the animal's general health. If there is a gum infection present, add additional vitamin C (500–3,000mg daily) and raw garlic to their food. Bonemeal powder (⅛–½ teaspoon) added to food gives extra calcium and phosphorus for healthy teeth.

Aromatherapy – Lavender and peppermint oils can be used externally for massaging inflamed or sore gums.

Biochemical tissue salts – Use calc. flour. to strengthen teeth.

Herbs – Echinacea and goldenseal tincture can be used directly on gums. They can also be taken in food to help boost the immune system.

Homoeopathy – Use apis. mel. for swollen gums, hepar. sulph. for infected gums that bleed easily and smelly breath. Merc. sol. is a good all-round remedy for gum disease.

Travel sickness

Most pets have no trouble travelling in the car or on a train, but others can become anxious and fearful and some are physically sick. Bach flower remedies will help with fears and anxieties related to travel (see behavioural problems and chapter nine), whilst there are a few natural remedies that can help with physical sickness. If possible make sure your pet has access to fresh air while travelling.

Diet – A healthy diet generally will help to keep the digestive system in good condition. Do not feed your pet for at least an hour before travelling and make sure they have fresh water available at all times.

Aromatherapy – A few drops of peppermint or melissa on your pet's blanket while travelling can help.

Bach flower remedies – Rescue remedy is the best all-round remedy for travel sickness combined with scleranthus. Also see chapter nine for remedies relating to specific fears or anxieties.

Biochemical tissue salts – Use kali. phos. for nervous sickness, nat. phos. for stomach upsets.

Herbs – Ginger is probably the first choice for travel sickness, or try peppermint. Ginger can be added to homemade biscuits or given as tablets, capsules or tincture. Peppermint can be given as a tea or tincture half an hour before the journey.

Homoeopathy – Give cocculus at least half an hour before travelling. Give ipecac. for nausea and vomiting at least half an hour before travelling. Nelson's make a travel sickness tablet for animals.

Vomiting

Occasional vomiting in cats and dogs is quite normal, since they get upset stomachs just like us, but frequent or repeated vomiting is a sign of a more serious problem. Occasional vomiting can be caused by a number of things including fur balls, stomach upsets and food or plant material getting stuck in the throat. Sometimes animals intentionally eat grass to make themselves sick as a way of cleansing their system.

More serious cases of vomiting, which might bring up blood, can indicate an infection, worms, liver, kidney or pancreatic disease, poisoning or digestive problems, and should always be checked out by your vet.

Diet – The best treatment for a sick animal is to fast them for 24 hours to let their system clear of toxins. You can leave a bowl of vegetable broth water or rice water available for them to drink, as well as fresh drinking water (see fasting in chapter three). An animal that has been sick will often be dehydrated, so they need to have plenty of fluids. Once they begin to eat again, the first few meals should be bland and easy to digest. Add a good-quality multi-mineral and vitamin supplement to their food for a few weeks. Vomiting can rob the body of important nutrients and these need to be replaced. Use acidophilus powder to rebalance the internal environment.

Aromatherapy – Lavender or peppermint can be massaged into the abdomen or used in a diffuser/burner.

Bach flower remedies – Crab apple is the cleansing remedy. Use olive for physical exhaustion, hornbeam for fatigue and to help build up a sickly animal.

Biochemical tissue salts – Use ferr. phos. for vomiting undigested food, nat. sulph. for bile, combination S for stomach upsets.

Herbs – Slippery elm powder in food helps to soothe the stomach. Aloe vera juice is soothing and healing and provides nutrients. Chopped mint leaves can be added to their food or given as a tea.

Homoeopathy – Use nux vomica for occasional vomiting associated with stomach upset. Use phosphorus if they are sick immediately after food, arsen. alb. for vomiting with diarrhoea.

Weight problems

This includes loss of weight, being overweight, obesity.

OVERWEIGHT/OBESITY

Animals in the wild are rarely overweight, but it is a common problem with domestic pets. As many as 25–30 per cent of dogs are overweight; some are obese. Cats are less prone to becoming overweight; none the less, fat cats do exist! Overfeeding, allergies, constipation and incorrect diet are usually at the root of the problem, therefore diet is the most important thing to be looked at. There are other causes of weight gain, including heart disease, liver disease, kidney disease and an underactive thyroid, therefore it is best to get a vet's diagnosis first to eliminate more serious causes. Overweight animals are less healthy and more prone to illness than thinner animals, and obesity puts excessive strain on the heart and other organs and can lead to problems such as arthritis, rheumatism, diabetes and lowered immunity. Obese animals have a much shorter life expectancy.

Diet – Changing to a natural preservative-free or allergy diet is essential, and this may be enough on its own to return your pet to its optimum weight without reducing its food intake. Many commercial pet foods are high in sugars and fat and provide less than nutritious calories, which may cause your pet to overeat. Avoid giving lots of titbits and treats between meals and don't feed your pet from the table – this sets up bad habits which are hard for everyone to break! An overweight animal is often overloaded with toxins and has a sluggish eliminative system, so a day's fast on a weekly basis can really help in the first few months of treatment (see chapter three for dietary guidelines). Give a good-quality multi-mineral and vitamin supplement. Kelp tablets assist the metabolism and have a cleansing action on the body.

Exercise – Make sure your pet is getting regular exercise appropriate to its breed and age.

Herbs – Seaweed stimulates the metabolism and can be helpful with weight loss or an underactive thyroid. You can buy dried seaweed which can be cooked with a brown rice diet, or use kelp tablets. Aloe vera juice is a rich source of nutrients and an intestinal cleanser and helps relieve constipation. Dandelion and parsley help get rid of water retention.

UNDERWEIGHT

Weight loss can be caused by a number of things, including allergies, worms, inadequate digestion (malabsorption), incorrect diet, overactive thyroid, not enough food, cancer, liver disease, pancreatic disease, infections, emotional upsets such as loss or grief, or a major trauma like an operation. With cats, there is always the finicky eater syndrome to consider, and it may just take time and patience to introduce them to a new and healthier way of eating. As a first step it is always best to get a vet to check your pet for any serious underlying problems, especially if the weight loss happens suddenly.

Diet – Diet is the key to weight gain once any serious underlying problems have been addressed. Change your pet's diet to a natural preservative-free diet including plenty of raw food. The following foods can be added to their meal to encourage weight gain: oats (porridge), olive oil, sunflower oil or corn oil, goat's milk, goat or ewe's milk yoghurt, brewer's yeast, wheat germ, dried fruit and eggs. Cats can have butter added to their food as well. Watercress helps to promote digestion. Initially you may have to give your pet several small meals a day while you are building them up. Also give digestive enzymes, a good-quality multi-mineral and vitamin supplement and royal jelly capsules. In cases of inadequate digestion, alfalfa assists the absorption of nutrients (see chapter four).

Bach flower remedies – If your pet has gone off its food because it is grieving or stressed, flower remedies can help to rebalance their emotional state. Read chapter nine and choose one or more of the remedies that suit your pet's emotional state. Use beech for picky, finicky eaters, especially cats.

Herbs – Try using fenugreek seeds (½–3 teaspoons). These can be boiled up with brown rice or soaked in hot water overnight and the seeds and liquid added to food. Fenugreek smells of curry and your pet will too, but most cats and dogs love the taste! Fenugreek is a good digestive tonic.

EAR PROBLEMS

Ear problems are common in both cats and dogs and include ear mites (see parasites), discharge, wax, smelly ears, irritation, inflammation and infections.

Signs and symptoms of ear problems include frequent head shaking, scratching, clawing or pawing at the ears, rubbing the ears on the ground, discharge, heat, inflammation, irritation – and sometimes the ears can smell like sweaty socks or a ripe cheese!

Ear problems can be caused by a number of things, including grass seeds getting caught in the ear, allergies, injuries and infections (fungal, bacteria or yeast). Many of the flop-eared dogs, like spaniels and setters, are prone to ear infections because their ears are closed from the air, becoming a perfect environment for fungus and bacteria to multiply. If something gets stuck in the ear accidentally you must get your vet to remove it, since poking around in an animal's ear can damage it.

Ear problems can be cleared up very effectively using natural remedies, and the sooner the problem is caught the better. Left untreated, ear infections can spread to other areas of the body. Suitable treatments include acupuncture, aromatherapy, diet and food supplements, flower essences, healing, herbs and homoeopathy. Before treating your pet at home read the relevant chapters for information on treatment, remedies, dosage, suppliers, etc.

Diet – A preservative-free natural diet will enhance your pet's health and help to clear up infections and boost the immune system. Ear problems caused by allergies should also clear up once your pet is changed to an allergy-free diet. Vitamins A and E help to heal skin problems. Follow the diet and supplement recommendations in chapters three and four.

Apple cider vinegar or lemon juice in water can be used to clean out the ears of flop-eared dogs and help to fight against bacteria and infections. Check their ears regularly for grass seeds and infections and, to give their ears some fresh air, pin them back occasionally with a clothes peg.

Aromatherapy – Tea tree oil and garlic oil have anti-fungal and anti-bacterial properties and can be used with olive oil/sweet almond oil to clean out infected ears. Add a couple of drops of tea tree oil to two to three ounces of olive/almond oil and put this in the affected ear. Massage gently for a few minutes and then wipe the ear to remove any excess oil. This also helps to bring wax and sticky discharges to the surface and can dislodge foreign bodies that have got stuck. Almond oil and olive oil soften and dissolve dark waxy discharges and are soothing and healing. You can also add some vitamin E to the oil mixture, which is also soothing and healing.

Bach flower remedies – Use crab apple for cleansing and detoxifying, hawthorn for rundown animals.

Herbs – Aloe vera juice can also be used for cleaning and fighting infections and has a soothing effect on painful ears. Put two to three ounces of liquid into the affected ear, massage for a few minutes and then clean out any excess with cotton wool. Witch hazel is soothing and can be used to clean infected or inflamed ears.

Homoeopathy – Use hepar. sulph. for inflamed ears which are sensitive to touch, graphites for smelly discharges, rhus. tox. for chronic ear infections, hepar. sulph. for offensive smelly discharges, merc. sol. for suppurating ears with smelly discharge, silicea for recurrent ear infections. Calendula tincture can be diluted in warm water with sea salt to clean the ears. Calendula lotion can be used to soothe irritated or inflamed ears.

EYE PROBLEMS

Eye problems in cats and dogs should always be seen by a vet first so that you know what the trouble is. Depending on what is wrong, there is much that can be done for the eyes using natural therapies and remedies. Common eye problems include cataracts, conjunctivitis, injuries and failing eyesight. Suitable treatments for eye problems include acupuncture, aromatherapy, diet and food supplements, flower essences, healing, herbs and homoeopathy.

Before treating your pet at home, read the relevant chapters for information on treatment, remedies, dosage, suppliers, etc.

Cataracts

Cataracts are fairly common in older pets and are recognisable as a cloudy white or blue film over the eye which can eventually lead to blindness. They can be caused by injury, allergies, diabetes and infections, but many health professionals feel they are a result of internal toxins and malnutrition. Diet is a vital part of the healing process and a pet brought up on a natural diet will probably never have cataracts. In many cases, changing to a natural preservative-free diet will arrest the progress of cataracts.

Diet – Follow the guidelines for a natural preservative-free diet and supplement programme in chapters three and four, including vitamins A, C and E. Zinc is also a good mineral for eye health. Raw cucumber can be used over the eye or the juice used for bathing.

Bach flower remedies – Use crab apple to remove toxins.

Herbs – Aloe vera juice is a good internal cleanser and can also be used diluted as an eye wash. Eyebright can be used externally as an eye wash or taken internally.

Homoeopathy – Silica delays the progress of mature cataracts. Diluted cineraria tincture can be used as an eyedrop. Use calc. carb. for old, overweight pets.

Conjunctivitis

Conjunctivitis is an inflammation of the tissue around the eye and is common in both cats and dogs. The usual causes are something getting into the eye, allergy, infection or an irritant. Dogs that stick their heads out of car windows on journeys can get conjunctivitis if something flies into their eye. Signs of conjunctivitis are red, sore-looking eyes with a runny discharge.

Diet – Change to the natural preservative-free diet and supplement programme outlined in chapters three and four to keep your pet healthy and strong. Zinc is a good supplement for healing eye problems. Slices of cucumber held over the eye can cool hot, inflamed eyes, or the juice can be used as eyedrops.

Aromatherapy – Soak some cotton-wool in tepid water with a few drops of chamomile and hold over the eye.

Herbs – Tea made from eyebright or goldenseal can be used to bathe the eye. Vitamin E can be added to the liquid to enhance the healing process. A pad of cotton-wool soaked in witch hazel can be held over shut eyes. Eyebright and goldenseal can be taken internally as well.

Homoeopathy – Use euphrasia diluted in water for bathing the eye, apis. mel. for sudden attacks and swelling. Use euphrasia tablets for profuse watering, and argent. nit. for uncomplicated cases.

Injuries

Eye injuries are pretty common, resulting from fights, accidents, foreign bodies getting into the eye and bruising.

Diet – A good healthy diet and supplement programme will help with the healing process (see chapters three and four). Slices of cucumber can be held over the eye, or use the juice as an eyedrop.

Herbs – Eyebright can be used externally to clean the eye or taken internally. Cotton-wool soaked in witch hazel used externally is soothing.

Homoeopathy – Arnica ointment can be used externally around the eye to reduce swelling or taken internally as tablets to reduce swelling. Calendula lotion externally can soothe and relieve pain.

Failing eyesight

Old age is often accompanied by failing eyesight and many older pets develop cataracts (see above). There is little you can do to prevent naturally degenerating eyesight; however, the Bach flower remedies can help your pet adapt to change and cope with progressive loss of sight, especially if they become nervous or fearful with it (see chapter nine).

IMMUNE SYSTEM AND INFECTIOUS DISEASES

An animal's immune system protects it from infectious diseases like kennel cough and distemper. A healthy immune system will be able to defend the animal against viral, bacterial or fungal invasions, whereas a weakened immune system will not. This is a key point in understanding why some animals become infected and others do not, since infectious agents are always around, but only those with weakened defence systems become ill.

Many of the infectious diseases that affect cats and dogs can be fatal, therefore it is vital to take your pet to the vet if you suspect an infection. Some of the more common infectious diseases include parvovirus, distemper, kennel cough, lyme disease, canine hepatitis, feline leukaemia virus, feline infectious peritonitis, feline immunodeficiency virus, chlamydia (cats), ringworm, skin diseases, wound infections, auto-immune diseases (allergies, asthma) and cancer.

Many things can weaken the immune system and leave a pet open to disease, including stress, chemicals and food additives, heavy-metal poisoning, air pollution, frequent or multiple vaccinations, bad diet and unnatural lifestyle. Our pets are getting diseases now that were unheard of 100 years ago, and many people put this down to increased stress on the immune system. The best way to fight infection is to keep the immune system strong – prevention is better than cure. Pets that are fed a natural preservative-free diet and regular supplements are far less likely to become infected, and far more likely to recover if they do become ill.

Signs that your pet has an infectious illness are runny, watery eyes, coughing, sneezing, loss of appetite, listlessness, vomiting, diarrhoea and a fever. The earlier the infection is caught, the easier it is to cure.

Natural treatments and remedies are highly effective in boosting and strengthening the immune system and maintaining resistance to infectious diseases. However, always take your pet to see the vet, since infectious diseases can be fatal. Let them know what natural treatment approach you wish to follow and get a referral. Suitable treatments include acupuncture, aromatherapy, diet and food supplements, flower essences, healing, herbs and homoeopathy.

Before treating your pet at home, read the relevant chapters for information on treatment and remedies, dosage, suppliers, etc.

Diet – A natural preservative-free diet and supplements is the cornerstone of a healthy immune system, whereas a bad diet invites disease. Fasting is really helpful when there is a fever or at the onset of an infection (see chapter three for details). If you only add one supplement make it vitamin C. It helps to rebuild the immune system and is a good preventative measure against infections. Use high quantities of vitamin C spread throughout the day (you can go to bowel-tolerance levels). Other immune-boosting supplements are B-complex vitamins, vitamins A and D (or use cod liver oil), zinc, magnesium, calcium, Vitamin E and selenium. Apple cider vinegar added to food or water is also an immune booster, as is royal jelly. Do not use brewer's yeast in cases of fungal or bacterial infections (see chapter four for details on food supplements).

Aromatherapy – Immune-boosting oils include lemon, sage, thyme, tea tree and bergamot. They can be used for massage or in a diffuser. Use bergamot, lemon and eucalyptus for fevers. Using essential oils in a diffuser/burner can help to prevent the spread of infections to other animals.

Bach flower remedies – Use rescue remedy at the onset of symptoms, crab apple for cleansing, hornbeam to strengthen, olive for very ill, weak animals. There are many other potent flower essences from around the world that are helpful in fighting infections (see 'Further reading', chapter nine).

Herbs – Use goldenseal and echinacea for the immune system. Garlic has anti-viral, anti-bacterial and anti-fungal properties. St John's wort has reputed anti-viral properties. Aloe vera is a liver cleanser and digestive aid. Other liver-supportive herbs are dandelion, parsley and red beet powder. Nutritious herbs include alfalfa, oatstraw, horsetail, ginseng and liquid chlorophyll.

Homoeopathy – Use aconite at the start of symptoms, belladonna for fevers, gelsemium for flu-like symptoms or distemper.

The kidneys, bladder and urinary tract make up the urinary system, which can be prone to bacterial infections and degenerative disease. It is crucial that the urinary system stays healthy, since it is responsible for removing waste products from the body, particularly the by-products of protein metabolism. Protein in the urine is a sure sign that there is something wrong with the kidneys. Some of the more common problems affecting cats and dogs are cystitis, bladder and kidney stones, kidney disease and incontinence. Suitable treatments include acupuncture, aromatherapy, biochemical tissue salts, diet and food supplements, flower essences, healing, herbs and homoeopathy.

Before treating your pet at home, read the relevant chapters for information on the treatment, remedies, dosage, suppliers, etc.

Bladder/kidney stones and gravel

Bladder and kidney stones are formed out of mineral salts and can cause intense discomfort to an animal. Inadequate diet and lack of fluids are the most common causes, therefore a good-quality natural diet is a simple preventative measure. Stones and gravel tend to form more often in the bladder than in the kidneys and cause recognisable symptoms like recurrent cystitis, incontinence and difficulty urinating. There may also be blood in the urine.

Much can be done with natural treatments and remedies to prevent stones from developing, especially with a foundation of a natural diet and supplement programme.

Diet – Change your pet's food to a natural preservative-free diet. Make sure they also have plenty of fresh water available, preferably filtered or bottled water. Dried food should never be given to pets with bladder or kidney stones, since it is thought to be a major contributing factor. The phosphorus content of the diet should be kept low, which means giving your pet good-quality protein (meat, fish, eggs, yoghurt, tofu and beans, but not red meat) and avoiding poor-quality protein such as meat by-products and meat derivatives. Add apple cider vinegar to their food or water to acidify the urine. An acid urine can dissolve gravel and small stones. Other positive foods include brown rice, potatoes, asparagus, carrots and oat flakes.

High quantities of vitamin C help to acidify the urine and dissolve stones. Vitamin C also detoxifies the body and reduces the likelihood of stones forming. Also give vitamin E, cod liver oil (or vitamins A and D), magnesium, calcium and vitamin B complex (see chapters three and four).

Aromatherapy – Use juniper, sandalwood and ylang ylang .

Bach flower remedies – Use crab apple for cleansing.

Biochemical tissue salts – Use mag. phos. and calc. phos. given together.

Herbs – Use couchgrass, uva ursi and sarsparilla. Parsley, nettle and dandelion are also helpful herbs.

Homoeopathy – Use calc. carb. for overweight animals, calc. phos. for lean animals.

Cystitis

Cystitis is an uncomfortable and painful infection of the urinary tract and tends to be more common in cats than in dogs. It has noticeable symptoms including an urgent need to urinate and frequent urination but not passing much. There can be a fever, and sometimes there is blood in the urine. Cystitis is often recurrent and if unchecked can lead to more serious kidney infections. It is usually caused by a bacterial infection (see immune system and infections) or bladder stones. Natural treatments and dietary changes can greatly help alleviate the problem and prevent recurrence.

Diet – Follow a natural preservative-free diet and supplement regime outlined in chapters three and four. Never feed dried foods to pets with cystitis. Cystitis is rare in animals that are fed a natural homemade diet. In acute cases, a day of fasting on barley water and parsley cleanses the system and fights bacteria. High levels of vitamin C given throughout the day at bowel-tolerance level will also help. (Also see bladder and kidney stones.)

Aromatherapy – Use juniper, tea tree, sandalwood and bergamot.

Bach flower remedies – Use rescue remedy.

Biochemical tissue salts – Use kali. mur., kali. phos. and mag. phos.

Herbs – Use horsetail, uva ursi and nutrient herbs, such as dandelion, parsley, watercress and nettles. Unsweetened cranberry juice acidifies the urine and makes it difficult for bacteria to thrive.

Homoeopathy – Use cantharis for acute cystitis.

Feline Urology Syndrome (FUS)

The symptoms are similar to cystitis (including depression, loss of appetite, straining to pass urine) and should be checked out by your vet. It is caused by tiny crystals blocking the flow of urine from the bladder, which can lead to cystitis and even kidney failure. Never feed dried foods to a cat with FUS. This is because the protein quality in dried foods is low and this causes the urine to be alkaline. An alkaline urine encourages the growth of unfriendly bacteria and the formation of stones and gravel. (Also see cystitis and bladder and kidney stones.)

Incontinence

It is a very upsetting experience for pets to be incontinent as they don't like upsetting their owners by urinating in the home or missing the litter tray. Incontinence is usually a symptom of bladder or kidney infection, and these should be checked out first. Incontinence can sometimes have an emotional problem at its root (see behavioural problems). It tends to affect older cats and dogs and can be caused by spaying and repeated infections like cystitis.

Diet – Follow the guidelines for a natural preservative-free diet with no dry foods, milk, organ meat or yeast. Include raw vegetables in their food, e.g. carrots, green beans, asparagus. Apple cider vinegar adds potassium. Barley water and honey assist urinary function (also see bladder and kidney stones). Also give B complex, vitamin C, cod liver oil (or vitamins A and D), vitamin E, zinc, calcium and magnesium (see chapters three and four).

Aromatherapy – Use juniper.

Bach flower remedies – Use hornbeam for strengthening.

Herbs – Use parsley, nettles, dandelions, horsetail.

Homoeopathy – Use causticum for weak bladder muscles, calc. flour. for young animals, apis for pets that cannot make it outside or to the litter, sulphur for incontinence and frequency.

Kidney disease

The main function of the kidneys is to eliminate waste, maintain the body's fluid balance and control blood pressure. Kidney problems are fairly common in older cats and dogs, particularly kidney failure which is slow and progressive.

Signs and symptoms of kidney disease are gradual weight loss, lethargy, lack of appetite, bad breath, increased thirst (cats normally drink very little unless on a dry-food diet), poor coat condition, smelly coat, inability to hold urine overnight and vomiting. Repeated bouts of cystitis can eventually lead to kidney disease, which is one of the leading causes of death in cats. Skin problems are often associated with kidney disease and can precede later kidney failure.

Always take your pet to the vet if you suspect kidney disease, as it can be serious if not treated. Natural medicine has a lot to offer, especially in the area of nutrition.

Diet – Natural treatment involves helping the kidneys to do their job, therefore the fewer toxins there are in your pet's diet, the less strain there will be on the kidneys. Change to a natural preservative-free diet and supplement regime. Cut out all salt and excess phosphorus. (If you are buying ready-made food then check the labels to determine phosphorus and sodium content.) The protein content of your pet's diet should also be low, but make sure it is good-quality protein, i.e. not meat by-products, meat derivatives, etc. Do not use dried food, as this can lead to dehydration and the low protein quality of dried food can lead to cystitis, FUS and kidney and bladder stones.

Fresh filtered or bottled water should be available at all times. Barley water with some honey added is also a good kidney cleanser. Other helpful foods for the kidneys are potatoes, green beans, asparagus, parsnips (raw, grated) and green leafy vegetables. Supplement the diet with B complex, vitamin C, cod liver oil (or vitamins A and D), calcium and magnesium. Apple cider vinegar added to water or food adds potassium. Also give small amounts of corn oil or safflower oil, and a good-quality multi-mineral and vitamin supplement (see chapters three and four).

Aromatherapy – Use juniper and bergamot.

Bach flower remedies – Use olive for weak, exhausted animals, crab apple for cleansing.

Biochemical tissue salts – Nat. mur. helps with fluid balance.

Herbs – Nettles and parsley are gentle diuretics and help the kidneys remove waste. Couch grass, horsetail and uva ursi are also helpful for the kidneys. Alfalfa adds a wide range of nutrients.

Homoeopathy – Use nux vomica to reduce toxicity, phosphorus for acute kidney disease with vomiting, nat. mur. for increased thirst and poor skin condition.

MUSCLE AND JOINT PROBLEMS

Muscle and joint problems include arthritis, rheumatism, hip dysplasia, bone fractures, sprains and strains, dislocation, slipped discs, spinal problems and paralysis. Suitable treatments include acupuncture, aromatherapy, biochemical tissue salts, chiropractic, diet and supplements, flower essences, healing, herbs, homoeopathy, osteopathy and T-touch.

Before treating your pet at home, read the relevant chapters for information on treatment, remedies, dosage, suppliers, etc.

Arthritis (osteoarthritis and rheumatism)

Arthritis is an inflammation of the joints, mostly affecting older pets, and can be crippling and extremely painful. The two most usual forms of the disease are osteoarthritis and rheumatism. Dogs tend to be affected more than cats.

Signs and symptoms of arthritis in your pet include stiffness, especially after rest, aggravated symptoms in cold, damp weather, difficulty jumping up or climbing stairs, lagging behind on walks, soreness hours after exercise, swollen or painful joints and lameness.

Nutrition is the key element in the holistic prevention and treatment of arthritis to the extent that animals brought up on a natural preservative-free diet seldom suffer from this disease. Arthritis is often a result of poor nutrition combined with hereditary factors.

Arthritis is a whole-body disease and therefore needs an holistic approach to treatment. Because it is an auto-immune disease, emphasis is on boosting the immune system and improving the overall health of the animal as well as encouraging elimination of toxins. Toxins settle in the joints, making the problem worse, therefore detoxification needs to be part of treatment. Holistic treatment may not bring about a complete cure, but it can slow down progression and give your pet a much more comfortable life. Arthritis is a chronic disease, therefore natural therapies require patience and commitment since treatment will be long-term.

Structural therapies like chiropractic and osteopathy are of great help in all musculo-skeletal problems. Acupuncture and healing also help greatly with pain relief, boosting the immune system and stimulating self-healing. If you do decide to opt for the natural approach, remember that medical drugs should only be phased out under veterinary guidance.

Diet – Change to a natural preservative-free diet which includes plenty of raw vegetables and fruit, easily digested protein, e.g. fish, eggs, chicken, turkey, live yoghurt, cottage cheese and tofu, cooked whole grains, e.g. brown rice, and pure fresh water, not tap water. Fasting for one day a week helps to remove toxins from the system. During the fast you can give your pet carrot and celery juice, barley water, rice water or vegetable broth water. If your pet is overweight it puts extra strain on joints and ligaments and speeds up degeneration (see weight problems/overweight).

Other helpful additions to the diet include apple cider vinegar (½–3 teaspoons), a yeast-free vitamin B complex (1–3 tablets), kelp (1–3 tablets), vitamin C (500–7,000mg), cod liver oil (½–3 teaspoons), vitamin E (50–300iu), bonemeal, wheat germ oil (½–2 teaspoons), lecithin (½–2 teaspoons), and a good-quality pet multi-mineral and vitamin complex. Older pets or those with digestive problems may also need digestive enzymes. As a preventative measure, it is really important to give good nutrition to pregnant females (to protect their young from developing arthritis) by providing a natural diet and additional vitamin C (see chapter four).

Exercise – Ensure moderate, regular exercise related to your pet's breed and plenty of sunshine and warmth. Dogs benefit from swimming in the sea, but make sure they are dried well afterwards so that they do not sit around damp and cold.

Aromatherapy – Massaging the affected areas using essential oils is soothing to stiff and painful joints and increases the circulation. Beneficial oils include juniper, eucalyptus, birch, thyme, rosemary and pine. Add a few drops of one or more essential oils to a base of olive oil or sweet almond oil.

Bach flower remedies – Use crab apple for cleansing and detoxifying, hornbeam for strengthening.

Biochemical tissue salts – Use calc. flour., nat. phos., nat. sulph. Use silica for inherited joint pains, combination M for rheumatic pain.

Herbs – The following herbs help to cleanse and reduce inflammation: celery seeds, garlic, meadowsweet, devil's claw and cornsilk. Use skullcap, valerian and feverfew for pain relief. Alfalfa, aloe vera and chlorophyll help to cleanse toxins from the body. Use echinacea and goldenseal for the immune system.

Liquorice root is a natural anti-inflammatory. Other herbs that can be added to food include the green leaf herbs, such as nettles, dandelions, watercress and parsley, which are all good detoxifiers.

(Parsley and watercress are also high in vitamin C.) Comfrey is the bone-healing herb.

A combination of slippery elm and cayenne in a 10:1 ratio can be mixed into a paste with water and used as a poultice.

Homoeopathy – Rhus. tox. is the 'classic' arthritis remedy for stiffness on getting up which eases with movement but is worse in cold, damp weather. Use bryonia when pain is worse for movement, arnica for swelling or bruising, calc. carb. for old, stiff, overweight pets.

Broken bones and fractures

Broken bones and fractures are usually caused by accidents, particularly being hit by a car, but they can also be caused by brittle bone disease (osteoporosis). Osteoporosis is a thinning of the bones usually caused by inadequate diet or kidney disease. As the bones become more brittle it leaves the animal susceptible to fractures and breaks.

The signs and symptoms will be pretty obvious, especially if the fracture has penetrated the skin. Other signs include misshapen bones and joints, swelling and lameness.

Fractures and breaks need immediate veterinary attention. If you have the Bach flower rescue remedy or homoeopathic aconite to hand, give one or both to reduce the shock and trauma. Once the bones have been reset, natural remedies and treatments can speed up the healing process and support recovery. Acupuncture, McTimoney chiropractic and osteopathy are particularly helpful in treating broken bones and fractures.

Diet – A good-quality diet and supplements regime will help to heal bones and speed recovery. Give plenty of vitamin C (double dose) and bonemeal (see chapters three and four for details).

Bach flower remedies – Give rescue remedy for shock and trauma.

Biochemical tissue salts – Use calc. flour. and calc. phos. given together.

Herbs – Comfrey is known as the 'bone-knitting' herb and can be taken internally or used externally as a poultice. Comfrey ointment can also be applied externally. Alfalfa, horsetail grass and oatstraw add calcium to the diet for bone-healing. A poultice of fresh mullein leaves can also be used.

Homoeopathy – Give aconite immediately for shock and trauma, arnica for bruising. Symphytum (comfrey) promotes healing and knitting of bones. Silicea strengthens the skeleton. Give calc. carb. for heavy, overweight animals, calc. phos. for thinner animals.

Hip dysplasia (dogs)

Hip dysplasia is a malformation of the hip's ball-in-socket joint. It affects one or both hips and can lead to a complete loss of use of the hind legs. It is particularly prevalent among large breeds of dogs like German shepherds, labradors and retrievers. As the dog gets older it also becomes more prone to arthritis and rheumatism in the affected legs.

Symptoms of hip dysplasia are stiffness, a wobbly gait while walking, sitting down a lot and generally being out of sorts. Although the causes are thought to be hereditary, many holistic vets feel that generations of inadequate diet (particularly a lack of vitamin C) is the main cause of hereditary hip dysplasia. Natural treatments can help to prevent the problem recurring in future generations and can ease the condition for dogs that are already suffering. Acupuncture, healing, chiropractic and osteopathy are all good treatments for hip dysplasia, along with dietary changes and a good supplement programme.

Diet – Change to a natural preservative-free diet as outlined in chapter three. Pregnant bitches and puppies need additional vitamin C (500–5,000mg for adults, 50–100mg for puppies under six months old) and bonemeal daily (see chapters three and four). Also see arthritis.

Aromatherapy – See arthritis.

Bach flower remedies – See arthritis.

Herbs – Use comfrey or white willow bark for pain relief (dogs only), alfalfa.

Homoeopathy – Use conium for advanced hip dysplasia, calc. carb. for fat, young dogs, calc. phos. for lean, thin dogs.

Joint dislocation

The most usual causes of dislocated joints are road traffic accidents or falls. Veterinary treatment is essential, but you can also give your pet the Bach rescue remedy or homoeopathic aconite as a first-aid measure to reduce shock and trauma.

Signs and symptoms of dislocated joints are usually easy to see, such as misshapen joints, lameness and stiffness around the joint.

Once the joint has been put back into place, natural remedies and treatments will help speed recovery. A pet with damaged joints is more prone to getting arthritis at a later date. Acupuncture, chiropractic and osteopathy are particularly good treatments. (Also see hip dysplasia and arthritis.)

Diet – A good-quality natural diet and supplement programme are vital for speedy recovery. Give vitamin C (double dose) to heal damaged tissues, glucosamine sulfate (300–1,000mg) for cartilage and joint repair and maintenance of healthy joints, bonemeal for added calcium (see chapters three and four).

Bach flower remedies – Use rescue remedy as a first-aid measure for shock and trauma.

Biochemical tissue salts – Use calc. flour. and calc. phos. together.

Herbs – Alfalfa, comfrey, horsetail grass, oatstraw and kelp will all help with joint-healing and recovery.

Homoeopathy – Use aconite as a first-aid measure for shock and trauma, arnica for bruising, hypericum for pain relief.

Paralysis and spinal disease (spondylosis, spondylitis, slipped disc)

Spinal diseases and accidents involving the spine often lead to paralysis. Spinal diseases include spondylosis, spondylitis and slipped disc and are more common in dogs than in cats. They tend to be degenerative, becoming more apparent with age.

Breeds of dog with long bodies and short legs, such as bassett hounds and dachshunds, are particularly prone to spinal problems, as are some larger breeds like German shepherds. In cats, spinal problems are usually related to accidents, especially car accidents.

Spondylitis is a degenerative disease of the spine that causes pain and inflammation and is essentially arthritis of the vertebrae (see also arthritis). As it progresses, there is increased bone formation and the joints fuse together causing curvature of the spine. This becomes a chronic condition known as spondylosis.

Slipped disc is caused by the degeneration of a disc which then presses on the spinal cord, causing severe weakness and paralysis.

Accidents or diseases affecting the spine can also cause partial paralysis, usually of the hind quarters.

Some of the causes of spinal problems other than accidents are inadequate diet, lack of exercise and stress. There is, therefore, much that can be done as a preventative measure. Signs and symptoms include rigidity of the spine, pain on getting up, progressive paralysis of the back legs, loss of strength on the rear end, muscle wasting, curvature of the spine and loss of control of the bladder or bowels. Acupuncture, chiropractic and osteopathy are strongly recommended.

Diet – A good-quality diet and supplement programme is essential for keeping the musculo-skeletal system healthy (see arthritis and chapter three for details). Vitamin C (high dose) strengthens connective tissue, cartilage and bone. Also give vitamin E (300–600iu) and use castor oil as a compress for pain and swelling (see chapter four).

Exercise – Light exercise is important if the animal can manage. Swimming is a good way to exercise the body.

Aromatherapy – Lightly massage with the following oils: lavender, marjoram and rosemary.

Biochemical tissue salts – Use silica.

Bach flower remedies – Use hornbeam and olive to strengthen weak animals, rescue remedy and star of Bethlehem for injury.

Herbs – Use skullcap, valerian and feverfew for pain relief and as a relaxant. Use white willow (dogs only) for inflammation, alfalfa, horsetail grass and oatstraw for bones and joints, comfrey and skullcap to repair nerves and relieve pain.

Homoeopathy – Use nux vomica for slipped discs, pains, spasms and paralysis, arnica for swelling or bruising, ruta. grav. for slipped discs or injuries affecting the vertebrae, conium maculatum for rear-end paralysis.

Sprains and strains

Most active pets are likely at some time to suffer from sprains or strains, such as pulled or torn muscles, overworked muscles, stretched ligaments or swollen tendons. Signs of this in your pet include limping, holding up a paw, localised swelling and signs of pain.

Diet – A good-quality diet and supplement regime helps to promote healing and speeds recovery. Additional vitamin C helps to heal tissue and reduce inflammation. Calcium and magnesium help to reduce muscle spasms and pain. Fasting for 24 hours on just honey water also promotes healing (see chapters three and four).

Aromatherapy – Massaging the affected area with one or more of the following oils will ease pain and reduce inflammation and stiffness: birch, lavender, eucalyptus, juniper, rosemary.

Bach flower remedies – Use rescue remedy for shock.

Biochemical tissue salts – Use ferr. phos. or combination I for rheumatic pain.

Herbs – Comfrey can be taken internally or used as a cold compress. Alfalfa, horsetail and oatstraw add calcium for strains. Witch hazel can be used as a compress. Use herbal creams externally, such as arnica for bruising, ruta for injury to ligaments, and rhus. tox. for injury to muscles with swelling and stiffness. Tiger balm used externally also soothes sprains and strains.

Homoeopathy – Use arnica for bruising and pain, pulled tendons and ligaments with stiffness and pain. A cold compress of diluted arnica tincture is helpful in reducing swelling. Use rhus. tox. for persistent lameness and sore, stiff, swollen muscles, ruta. for injury, sprains and strains.

Parasites are creatures that live in or on your pet, such as worms and fleas. They are unwelcome lodgers, since they take as much as they can and give nothing back in return. Most pets at some time will be host to a parasitic invasion; however, healthy cats and dogs with a strong immune system are less likely to be bothered by parasites. A good natural diet and a healthy lifestyle are two of the most important front-line defences against these unwelcome guests.

Some of the most common parasites that affect dogs and cats are fleas, ticks, lice, mites and various kinds of worms. There is much you can do at home to prevent parasites in the first place, and natural treatments and remedies can help to eliminate the problem. Although there are plenty of chemically prepared flea powders and flea collars on the market, these contain harmful elements and repeated use can harm your pet. Suitable treatments include acupuncture, aromatherapy, biochemical tissue salts, diet and supplements, flower essences, healing, herbs and homoeopathy.

Before treating your pet at home, read the relevant chapters for information on treatment, remedies, dosage, suppliers, etc.

Ear mites

Ear mites live in an animal's ear canal and cause inflammation, irritation and a thick, brownish-red crust. They are common in cats and dogs and often spread from one to the other. Signs to look out for are lots of head shaking, along with excessive scratching and rubbing of their ears. Use a torch and check their ears for a dry, crumbly brown discharge inside the ear canal.

See fleas for general advice on treatment at home.

Specific treatment – Olive oil with vitamin E added can be poured into the ear and massaged for a while to loosen any crusty material and bring it to the surface. After a few minutes clean out the ear with cotton-wool. You can also clean the ear with garlic water (fresh garlic boiled in water, strained and cooled) or tea tree oil on the end of a cotton-wool bud. Never stick anything hard inside the ear. Clean the ears every day for at least a week. If the ears are very red and inflamed, calendula cream will help to soothe them. Also clean around the ears with herbal shampoo and use a herbal flea powder. Crab apple Bach flower remedy will help to expel impurities.

Homoeopathy – Use sulphur for hot, red, smelly ears.
If the mites persist, consult your vet.

Fleas

Although fleas can affect any pet, the healthier it is the less likely it is to become infested. Fleas prefer animals in poor health with lowered immune systems and are usually only a nuisance in warm weather. During the summer months check your pet regularly for fleas. Apart from being able to see them, other signs to look out for are scratching, chewing and biting, licking their coat and pulling out hair. Some animals may have an allergic reaction to flea bites or have red and sore skin. Sometimes you can see flea dirt, which is dry, black and dust-like, on light-coloured animals.

Tapeworms are carried by fleas, so if your pet is infested with fleas they may also have worms.

Diet – A natural preservative-free diet will improve your pet's general health and enhance its immune system. Raw garlic is one of the best anti-parasite treatments – chop it up and put it in your pet's food or use garlic tablets/capsules if they don't like the taste (one clove for cats and small dogs, two cloves for medium dogs and three cloves for large dogs). Brewer's yeast is also a good repellant. This can be mixed into their food (one teaspoon daily for cats and small dogs, two teaspoons for medium dogs and three teaspoons for large dogs). Both garlic and brewer's yeast should be given for at least four weeks. Brewer's yeast can also be rubbed into your pet's coat and used as a natural flea powder. Give zinc (5–20mg daily) to help boost the immune system and vitamin C (500–5,000mg daily) to detoxify and boost the immune system. Use a yeast-free B-complex supplement if your pet is allergic to brewer's yeast (see chapters three and four).

Environment – If you find fleas on your cat or dog you can be sure that ten times that number are hiding in its environment! Eggs and larvae need to be eliminated as well, so flea control means cleaning and vacuuming all the places where your pet sleeps and lies. Regular cleaning and grooming interrupts the flea's life-cycle and makes breeding more difficult.

Aromatherapy – Lavender, lemon and peppermint deter fleas, and you can spray a mixture of essential oil, vodka and water on to your pet's bed or its fur as a deterrent. Other useful oils include eucalyptus, cedar, cypress and lemon. These can be massaged into their coat in a base oil and then combed through with a flea comb. You can add a few drops of oil on your pet's collar for a homemade natural flea collar.

Bach flower remedies – Use crab apple for cleansing.

Herbs – Mint leaves, lavender seeds, rosemary and sage can be left in and around your pet's bed to deter fleas. Goldenseal and echinacea taken internally will help to boost the immune system. Garlic taken regularly also helps to expel parasites (see diet). You can buy herbal flea powders or make up your own by mixing together powdered herbs like wormwood, eucalyptus, mint, rosemary, sage and yellow dock. Ask your herbalist to make up a powder for you. This can be rubbed into your pet's fur and combed through every day for about four weeks or until all the fleas have gone. (Remember to do this outside so that escaping fleas remain outside!) Garlic powder can also be rubbed into their fur.

Homoeopathy – Use pulex for flea allergies and flea infestation, sulphur where the skin is dry and flaky, and for scratching.

Grooming – Regular grooming is essential where external parasites are concerned. Get a special flea comb from the pet shop and thoroughly groom your pet from head to toe. (Again, remember to do this outside!) Essential oils and herbal flea powders can be combed into the fur at the same time.

Bathing – Bathing helps to prevent infestation and gets rid of existing fleas. There are natural pet shampoos on the market, or you could use washing-up liquid, garlic water or lemon water. (Garlic and lemon water are easily made by boiling crushed cloves of fresh garlic and/or a whole lemon in water and allowing it to cool.) Make sure you wash really well around the head and ears, which is where fleas tend to live. Keeping your pet clean and well groomed is essential when dealing with external parasites.

Lice

Lice are tiny insects which can be seen on the animal's fur – as can their eggs. A pet with lice will be restless and will rub and scratch its skin. Follow the treatment recommendations for fleas.

Mange

This is caused by tiny mites which burrow into the animal's skin. It is mostly found in dogs, but can affect cats too. Mange is a sign that the animal's immune system is under par. These parasites are difficult to remove and need veterinary guidance; however, follow the advice given for fleas to help boost your animal's general health, speed up their recovery and prevent recurrence. Also see immune system.

Ticks

Ticks are temporary parasites which burrow into the skin of warm-blooded animals to feast on their blood. They vary in size, from a few millimetres in length to a centimetre long when fully swollen with blood. Only the head end burrows into the skin and the body can easily be seen on the surface. Once they have eaten they usually fall off the host. However, tick bites can get infected, so it is best to remove ticks as soon as you notice them on your pet. (If they do get infected, follow the treatment advice for abscesses.)
See fleas for general treatment.

Removing a tick – Heat the end of a blunt knife in boiling water and press it on to the tick's body, being careful not to burn your pet's skin. The tick can then easily be pulled out with some tweezers. It is important to kill the tick before trying to get it out, otherwise its head can get left in and cause an infection.

Aromatherapy – Dab the tick with eucalyptus oil or camphor and then wait about a minute before pulling the tick out. Always make sure the whole tick is removed. Tea tree oil can be dabbed on the wound to prevent infection and to help the skin heal.

Worms

The two most common types of worm that affect cats and dogs are roundworm and tapeworm. They both live in the intestinal tract and can be seen in the faeces. Roundworms look like coiled springs and can also be seen in an animal's vomit, especially with young animals. Tapeworms are flat and segmented and the segments look like grains of white rice in the faeces or around the anus. Tapeworms can be carried by fleas, so a flea-infested animal should also be checked for tapeworm.

Pets most at risk from worms are newborn kittens and puppies (they can be passed from the mother), pets infested with fleas, animals that eat wild creatures and pets that are old or rundown.

Apart from seeing worms in the faeces, other signs that your pet has worms are weight loss, excessive appetite or lack of appetite, bad breath, bloated abdomen, bony body, vomiting, irritation around the anus, diarrhoea and a general decline in health.

Diet – Diet is one of the most important factors in treating worms.

PARASITES

The healthier your pet is, the more resistant it will be to a parasitic infestation. Change to a natural preservative-free diet. One of the most potent treatments is raw garlic added daily to food (½–2 cloves, depending on the animal's size). Other beneficial foods that can be added to meals include ground pumpkin or sesame seeds (¼–2 teaspoons), dried coconut (½–2 teaspoons), grated carrots (½–2 teaspoons), dried figs (1–3 figs, chopped), oat bran (½–2 teaspoons) and psyllium husks powder – roughage helps to carry worms out of the intestines. Fasting your pet for a day or two at the beginning of treatment is also helpful.

Pets with worms will be deficient in nutrients, so get them on to a good multi-mineral and vitamin formula. Make sure this contains zinc, iron, vitamin B complex, vitamin A and vitamin C. Vitamin C is a great detoxifier and can be given in addition to a multi-nutrient formula (500–5,000mg daily) (see chapters three and four).

Bach flower remedies – Use crab apple for cleansing, hawthorn for vitality.

Herbs – Use aloe vera, garlic, parsley, wormwood, black walnut hull and cloves.

Dr Hulda Clark's herbal parasite cure for pets:

1. Parsley water: Cook a big bunch of fresh parsley in four pints of water for three minutes. Throw away the parsley. Freeze most of the parsley water in small containers for later use. Put ½–2 teaspoons of parsley water on your pet's food daily.

2. Black walnut hull tincture: Use one week later, putting one drop on the food. Treat cats only twice a week; treat dogs daily (1–3 drops).

3. Wormwood capsules: One week after the black walnut tincture start the wormwood. Open the capsule and put a tiny pinch on their food every day, using a bigger pinch for large dogs.

4. Cloves: Begin this one week after the wormwood. Put a tiny pinch on their food, or a bigger pinch for large dogs.

By the fourth week your pet will be having parsley water, black walnut hull tincture, wormwood and cloves daily. Keep this up for another three to four weeks. If they get reinfested then repeat the regime from the beginning. The parasite cure can be given to your pet annually as a preventative measure. (This parasite cure for pets is taken from *The Cure for All Diseases* by Hulda Regehr Clark, PhD, N.D.; ProMotion Publishing.)

Homoeopathy For roundworms, use cina or chenopodium. For tapeworms, use granatum, Felix mas.

If you are unsure about whether your pet has worms or what type they are, consult your vet. Natural worming should only be done with your vet's knowledge, and if the problem does not clear up in three to four weeks you may need to consider conventional treatment, despite its toxic effects. Always get worming treatment from your vet specifically for your pet – do not buy them from supermarkets. Conventional wormers can do a lot of harm if they are not used properly and should never be used unless there is an actual infestation. Once your pet has been wormed, get their faeces checked again to make sure all the parasites have gone. As a daily preventive treatment, use raw garlic, oat bran or psyllium husks, raw carrots, beetroot or turnips, ground pumpkin seeds or sesame seeds, wheat germ oil (¼–1 teaspoon) and dried figs (see chapters three and four).

PREGNANCY AND ASSOCIATED PROBLEMS

Pregnancy is a time of high nutritional need when the animal requires not only more food but also a good, well-balanced supplement regime. If the female is in peak health there is a much better chance that all the offspring will be healthy and the pregnancy and labour problem-free. Nutrition is the most important factor in keeping your pet healthy throughout the pregnancy. Natural treatments can also help to alleviate problems that do arise, such as false pregnancy, inadequate milk production, infertility and mastitis.

There are plenty of good books detailing the ins and outs of breeding; this section is only aimed at listing the remedies and treatments that can positively assist pregnancy. Please read others books for advice on breeding.

Suitable treatments include acupuncture, aromatherapy, biochemical tissue salts, chiropractic, diet and supplements, healing, herbs, homoeopathy, osteopathy and T-touch.

Before treating your pet at home, always read the relevant chapters for information on treatment, remedies, dosage, suppliers, etc.

Many of the commonly used essential oils and herbs should not be used during pregnancy, so always be sure which ones are safe to use when treating your pet at home.

Abortion
See pregnancy.

False pregnancy
With a false pregnancy, a bitch can have all the symptoms of a real pregnancy without actually being pregnant. The signs are easily recognisable, including excessive hunger, swelling of the abdomen, milk production, restlessness – and she may go as far as making a nest for herself. Some dogs even take things into their nest to look after and can be quite aggressive if you try to take away her 'phantom pups'. The most common cause of a false pregnancy is hormonal imbalance.

Diet – A good-quality diet and supplement programme helps to bring the body back into balance (see chapters three and four). Evening primrose oil can also be added to their food.

Bach flower remedies – Use holly for aggression, mustard for mood swings, walnut to help them adapt to change.

Herbs – Use wild yam, chaste tree or motherwort.
Homoeopathy – Use sepia for aggressive or moody females, pulsatilla for symptoms that vary.

Inadequate milk production

Sometimes the female is not producing enough milk, or there may be no milk flow at all, which leaves a litter of hungry pups waiting to be fed. This can be caused by a hormonal imbalance, stress or mastitis (also see mastitis). Natural treatments and remedies can help to stimulate milk production and bring the body back into balance.

Diet – Chicken, oats and artichokes (artichoke hearts can be bought in tins or jars) have milk-stimulating properties and can make up a large proportion of the animal's meal. For general advice on nutrition and supplements, follow the dietary recommendations given for pregnancy (see chapters three and four).

Herbs – Fennel, milk thistle and fenugreek seeds stimulate milk production.

Homoeopathy – Pulsatilla can be given during labour to help stimulate milk production or after labour if there is inadequate milk.

Infertility

Infertility can be caused by a number of factors, including poor diet, nutrient deficiencies, hormonal imbalance, stress, heavy toxic load, obesity, problems with the reproductive organs – and, of course, unsuccessful mating or infertility in the stud dog or tom-cat.

A good-quality diet and supplement programme is fundamental to a healthy animal and can be enough on its own to turn round infertility, since nutrient deficiencies are a common cause. Structural causes may also be a part of the problem, therefore you might want to consider chiropractic or osteopathy as well.

Things to avoid prior to pregnancy are X-rays, steroid drugs, vaccines and antibiotics.

Diet – Change to a preservative-free natural diet, using as many organically grown ingredients as possible and fresh bottled or filtered water, not tap water (see chapter three for details). Add a higher dose than usual of supplements including vitamins A, C, D and B complex (or brewer's yeast). Vitamin E is especially important when treating infertility. Also add zinc, magnesium, calcium and evening primrose oil. Ginseng and royal jelly are also helpful supplements (see chapter four).

Bach flower remedies – Use clematis for animals lacking in energy, hawthorn to strengthen.

Herbs – Use chaste tree and black cohosh to help normalise the hormonal picture. Raspberry leaf helps to strengthen the womb and reproductive system. Use alfalfa and kelp for their rich nutrient content.

Homoeopathy – Use sepia for unpredictable, aggressive animals, pulsatilla for quiet, shy animals.

Mastitis

Mastitis (swollen mammary glands) is caused by a bacterial infection and animals are most susceptible to it when they are producing milk. The infected breast will be hard, sensitive and often red or purple in colour. Other symptoms to look out for are abscesses, fever, loss of appetite and depression. (Also see infections and the immune system.)

Diet – Follow the guidelines for a natural preservative-free diet and supplement programme outlined in chapters three and four.

Aromatherapy – Chamomile, geranium, peppermint and rose can be used to make an oil and water compress and held on the affected areas.

Bach flower remedies – Use hornbeam for strengthening, crab apple for cleansing, mustard for depression.

Herbs – Comfrey, slippery elm and poke root can be used as a soothing poultice. Use echinacea to help fight infection, poke root for infections and to reduce inflammation, cleavers for swollen glands.

Homoeopathy – Use aconite on the first signs of mastitis, belladonna when there is also fever and redness, bryonia for hot, painful and hard breasts worse for touch or movement. Phytolacca is an all-purpose mastitis remedy.

Pregnancy

Pregnancy is a time of great nutritional need, and cats and dogs will require more food and a good supplement regime throughout. Good nutrition is the key to a successful pregnancy and trouble-free delivery. It helps to prevent birth defects, runt litters and complications during and after labour. Before deciding to breed from your female, make sure she is fit and well. Pre-pregnancy health is of the utmost importance for both the males and females to ensure a litter of strong and healthy offspring.

Diet – We have already seen how important diet can be. We know, for example, that vitamin C helps to protect against hip dysplasia in dogs, and garlic can prevent worms in newborn kittens and pups. During pregnancy, huge nutritional demands are made on the female and continual breeding without attention to diet and supplements can leave an animal depleted and nutrient-deficient. As the pregnancy progresses, give her several small meals throughout the day rather than one big one. Follow the dietary recommendations in chapter three, and give a little more food than usual. Avoid chemicals, preservatives and drugs, such as commercial flea powders and worming tablets. Fresh bottled or filtered water should be available at all times.

Give a good-quality multi-vitamin and mineral complex; again, give her a higher dose than usual, but in balance. Make sure the multi-formula includes vitamins A, B complex, C, D and E. Wheat germ oil is a good source of vitamin E, and cod liver oil provides vitamins A and D. You may have to add extra vitamins C and E on top of the multi-vitamin (1,000–7,000mg of vitamin C daily and 50–500iu vitamin E daily). Calcium, magnesium and zinc are also important minerals. Add vegetable oil (or butter for cats) and cod liver oil. Also add some of the amino acid taurine (500mg) to a cat's diet. The protein quantity can be slightly increased for both cats and dogs, making sure it is good-quality protein including eggs, goat's milk, liver, cottage cheese, yoghurt, meat and fish. Oats are good for exhaustion after labour and help to strengthen the body. Kelp, alfalfa, watercress and liquid chlorophyll are good sources of vitamins and minerals and can be added to the diet. The pregnant female may also need to have some digestive enzymes added to food to help with digestion as the pregnancy progresses (see chapter four for supplement dosage).

Aromatherapy – It is best to avoid essential oils during pregnancy. Post-labour, clary sage and jasmine help to ease the pain of the birth.

Bach flower remedies – Use rescue remedy during and after labour, oak for exhaustion. Clematis helps newborn puppies and kittens to wake up and breathe. Use walnut to help the mother adjust, crab apple for cleansing after the birth.

Herbs – Raspberry leaf is traditionally used during pregnancy and helps to make labour and delivery easier. Use nettles to strengthen and support the whole body (good source of iron and vitamin C). Post-labour, use comfrey and horsetail for healing, milk thistle, fenugreek and fennel to help the flow of milk if there is poor milk production. (Herbs to avoid during pregnancy include aloe vera, wormwood, juniper, sage and strong laxative herbs.)

Homoeopathy – Caulophyllum given three to four weeks before the birth can ease labour (one tablet daily). Use pulsatilla during labour to promote milk production, ease the birth and calm the mother. Use aconite for fear or shock, arnica for bruising and exhaustion.

RESPIRATORY SYSTEM

Respiratory problems range from a stuffy nose and a cough to cat flu and bronchitis. Although cats are more prone to these problems than dogs, when a lot of dogs are kept in a confined space, such as at boarding kennels or dog shows, they can catch an infectious cough called kennel cough. There are many causes of respiratory diseases (infections, allergies, asthma, heart disease, parasites) – some of which, such as kennel cough, are serious – so always get your pet checked out by a vet so that you know exactly what is wrong. Most minor respiratory diseases respond well to natural remedies and there is much you can do to relieve your pet's condition. The following are a few of the more common conditions which will benefit from natural treatment. Suitable treatments include acupuncture, aromatherapy, diet and supplements, flower essences, healing, herbs and homoeopathy.

Before treating your pet at home, always read the relevant chapters for information about the treatment, the remedies, dosage, suppliers, etc.

Cat flu
See immune system and infectious diseases, coughs, sneezing and nasal discharge.

Coughs
There are many types of cough and many underlying causes. Some coughs are dry (no mucus) and others wet (involving bringing up mucus). Coughing is the commonest symptom of respiratory problems and can be brought on by a range of things, including infections (viral, bacterial, fungal), allergies, irritants, heart disease, lung congestion and parasites. Many pets also suffer from the adverse effects of their owners smoking. The most common type of cough in dogs is kennel cough, which is an infectious viral disease. The dog may not appear to be ill other than having a harsh, dry cough which is persistent and irritating. Cats can have a similar harsh, dry type of cough which may indicate bronchitis. Less serious coughs may be a result of a cold and repeated infections show that their immune system is weak and needs a boost.

Diet – Fasting is one of the most beneficial treatments for dogs or cats with an infectious cough or any virus-based respiratory disease, such as kennel cough and cat flu (also see immune system and infectious diseases). Raw garlic is a wonderful anti-viral treatment and can be added to your pet's food or given in capsule form when fasting. Change your pet's diet to a natural preservative-free diet. Supplement the diet with vitamin A (10,000iu daily) to heal mucus membranes, vitamin C (500–5,000mg daily), vitamin E (50–100iu daily) and zinc (5–20mg daily) to boost the immune system. Cod liver oil on a daily basis is also helpful (see chapters three and four).

Aromatherapy – Eucalyptus is the main oil for respiratory diseases. In this case it is best used in a diffuser/burner placed near your pet twice a day for about 15 minutes. Other useful oils include tea tree, pine and myrrh.

Bach flower remedies – Use crab apple to cleanse, hornbeam to strengthen, olive to give physical strength to an exhausted animal.

Biochemical tissue salts – Use ferr. phos. for acute, dry coughs, kali. sulph. if it is worse in the evening, mag. phos. if it is worse for lying down or for convulsive bouts of coughing, combination J for all coughs.

Herbs – Use garlic, liquorice, coltsfoot, goldenseal, echinacea, sage, thyme. Garlic is a good all-round infection-fighter. Echinacea and goldenseal are good immune-boosters. You can also buy ready-made herbal cough mixtures from herbalists and health-food shops. These usually contain herbs like liquorice, comfrey, coltsfoot, slippery elm and mullein and can be given in the following dosage: cats and small dogs – infant's dose, medium dogs – child's dose, large dogs – adult's dose. You can mix cough mixture with some raw honey to make it more tasty for your pet.

Homoeopathy – Use arsen. alb. for harsh coughing that worsens at night, bryonia for dry coughing that worsens with movement, aconite at the onset of coughing to stop it progressing further.

Kennel cough
See immune system and infectious diseases and coughs.

Stuffy nose, runny nose, sinusitis, sneezing, colds, catarrh
Colds and nasal problems are usually caused by infections (bacterial or fungal), allergies (cigarette smoke, dust, house dust mites) and sometimes tumours. Apart from obvious symptoms like sneezing and mucus discharges, your dog or cat may shake their head a lot too and be generally out of sorts. Cats are more prone to catarrhal problems than dogs.

Diet – A natural diet free of preservatives is important. Garlic and onions help to destroy mucus and can be cooked and put in your pet's food. Raw grated beetroot and carrots help to cleanse the body. Ginger helps to eliminate mucus from the sinuses. Supplement the diet with vitamin C (500–5,000mg daily), vitamin A (10,000iu daily), vitamin E (10–100iu daily) and zinc (5–20mg daily) (see chapters three and four).

Aromatherapy – Use eucalyptus, olbas oil, tea tree, thyme. These are best used in a diffuser/burner and placed near your pet twice a day for at least 15 minutes at a time. This will help to clear the nasal cavities.

Bach flower remedies – Use olive for an exhausted, rundown animal, hornbeam for strengthening, crab apple for cleansing.

Biochemical tissue salts – Use combination Q for catarrhal sinus disorders, nat. mur. for watery, clear discharges, calc. flour. for thick, yellow discharges, combination J for flu-like symptoms.

Herbs – Use goldenseal, garlic, liquorice, comfrey, fenugreek.

Homoeopathy – Use gelsemium for sneezing, runny nose, fever and raw throat. Kali. bich. is a good remedy for catarrhal symptoms. Use pulsatilla for conjunctivitis with catarrhal symptoms.

SKIN AND COAT

Skin and coat problems are very common amongst dogs and cats and seem to be on the increase. Diet is one of the most important factors in skin diseases and poor coat conditions and should be the first thing that is looked at. Much can be done just by changing your pet's diet to a more natural one. In some cases, a day's fast on a weekly basis can help, since it gives the animal's system a rest and promotes the elimination of toxins. Skin complaints can sometimes be difficult to shift completely, but you can go a long way towards keeping things under control by using natural remedies and dietary changes.

The following are some of the more common skin and coat problems that your pet may encounter, many of which can be treated at home. If your pet is suffering or the condition is too serious for home treatment, consult your vet.

Suitable treatments include acupuncture, aromatherapy, biochemical tissue salts, diet and supplements, flower essences, healing, herbs and homoeopathy.

Before treating your pet at home it is important to read the relevant chapters on the treatments and remedies you have chosen for information on dosage, suppliers, etc.

Abscesses

An abscess is a small amount of pus trapped under the surface of the skin. Usually they form after a bite or wound heals over, trapping bacteria or dirt inside which then becomes infected. Signs of infection include a red, swollen area of the skin that feels hot to the touch. It is also painful. If the abscess is in your dog or cat's mouth, they may also be off their food and generally out of sorts. (Mouth abscesses should be checked out by a vet in case dental treatment is needed.)

In order to heal, an abscess needs to be burst so that the pus can escape, bringing the infected material with it, and then the wound should be thoroughly cleaned. To draw out the pus, use hot compresses three or four times a day for 15 minutes at a time using warm, salty water with a few drops of tea tree oil added. Use one teaspoon of sea salt to a cup of warm water.

Diet – A natural preservative-free diet will help enhance the animal's immune system and self-healing ability. A good-quality multimineral and vitamin supplement for cats or dogs should be taken daily, along with additional zinc and vitamin C to help with the healing process (see chapters three and four).

Aromatherapy – Tea tree and thyme can be dabbed on the affected area. Lavender can be used as a warm compress on the abscess. Raw honey can also be spread on the abscess.

Bach flower remedies – Use crab apple for cleansing.

Biochemical tissue salts – Use silica for an abscess ready to burst or that has already burst.

Herbs – Garlic and echinacea boost the immune system and will help with the healing process. Garlic, echinacea and goldenseal can be used as a warm compress. Comfrey is also an important infection-healing herb and can be used externally or taken internally. Liquid garlic can be used to clean around the abscess. This can be bought ready-made, or make your own by liquidising a clove of garlic in a cup of water.

Homoeopathy – Use hepar. sulph. if the abscess is discharging, apis. mel. for hot, red abscesses, merc. sol. for mouth abscesses, silicea to help a long-term abscess to heal.

Anal glands

The anal glands lie just below a dog and cat's anus and act as the animal's scent glands. Usually they empty every time your pet has a bowel movement. However, constipation or insufficient roughage in the diet can prevent this from happening and can lead to swollen, blocked and infected anal glands. Overweight or aged animals can also be prone to anal gland problems. Signs of this in your pet are excessive licking of their bottom, itchy anus, dragging their bottom along the ground or crying out during bowel movements. If your pet is in a lot of pain or the condition does not improve within a few days, consult your vet.

Diet – This is the primary treatment. Give your pet a natural additive-free diet with adequate roughage. You can add raw grated carrot to their food, or some chopped-up prunes or figs. Olive oil added to food also helps to lubricate the bowel. Raw garlic is an intestinal antiseptic and can be mixed in with their food, or use garlic capsules if they don't like the taste. Provide plenty of fresh water (see chapters three and four).

Bach flower remedies – Use crab apple for cleansing.

Biochemical tissue salts – Use silica for repeated anal gland problems, as it encourages the discharge of pus.

Herbs – Use aloe vera juice taken internally, or add raw garlic to their food. Soak fenugreek seeds in warm water overnight, then mix the seeds into their food and give them the liquid to drink. Many animals love the taste of curry and enjoy fenugreek in their food. If using a brown-rice-based diet, cook the seeds in with the rice. Diluted witch hazel can be dabbed on the glands if they are particularly swollen. Psyllium husks added to food adds natural vegetable fibre to the diet and can help to ease the problem.

Homoeopathy – Use hepar. sulph. for infected glands, silicea for repeated anal gland problems. Arnica may also help with inflammation and discomfort.

Exercise – Exercise is also important to help eliminate toxins from the body and keep the anal glands emptying properly.

Coat problems

Coat problems include hair loss, dull coat, unhealthy-looking coat, dandruff and coarse or matted coat.

The condition of your pet's coat tells you a lot about their general health. A dull coat is one of the first signs of deteriorating health, whilst actual hair loss is a sign that the deterioration is more serious. Hair loss can be all over the body or in small localised patches. Many factors can lead to hair loss or an unhealthy coat, including poor diet, parasites, hormonal problems, digestive problems, allergies, infections, weakened immune system and liver or kidney problems.

Diet – A good, healthy diet is the key to a healthy-looking coat. The first thing you need to do is change your pet's food to a natural additive-free or allergy diet. Grated raw carrot and beetroot help to cleanse the liver and kidneys. Add brewer's yeast regularly to their food for extra B vitamins (or yeast-free B-complex supplement if a yeast allergy is suspected). Oil of evening primrose or linseed oil and fish liver oil will also help restore the coat's shine. Apple cider vinegar mixed into the food adds potassium to the diet. Also give zinc (5–20mg daily), vitamin C (500–5,000mg daily) and a good-quality multi-mineral and vitamin supplement for dogs or cats (see chapters three and four).

Aromatherapy – Rosemary is invigorating and may be massaged into dull coats or directly on to bald patches where there is hair loss. (Put a few drops in a base oil such as olive oil or sunflower oil.) Other useful oils include lavender, thyme, tea tree and pine. Your local pet shop may also stock a natural herbal shampoo, such as seaweed and birch, which relieves surface skin problems and deters fleas and parasites. Tea tree and rosemary oils are good for dandruff treatment.

Bach flower remedies – Use crab apple for general cleansing and detoxifying.

Biochemical tissue salts – Use kali. sulph., nat. mur. and silica for hair loss, nat. mur. and kali. sulph. for dandruff.

Herbs – Use aloe vera, echinacea, garlic, nettle, dandelion and seaweed. Aloe vera juice and raw garlic taken internally are very cleansing. Aloe vera spray can be used externally. Seaweed or kelp tablets help thyroid function and restore health to the coat. Nettles and dandelions cleanse the system and support the kidneys and liver. Echinacea enhances the immune system.

Homoeopathy – Use arsen. alb. for dandruff, or try sulphur. Use nat. mur. for hair loss, arsen. alb. for hair loss with itchyness, lycopodium for elderly and balding pets, pulsatilla for hair loss related to female hormone problems.

Grooming – Both cats and dogs will benefit from regular grooming to stimulate hair growth.

Eczema and dermatitis

Symptoms include general itching and scratching, along with inflamed red sores on the skin which can become infected. In long-term, chronic cases the skin can become dry and scaly, or it may be greasy, and some of the animal's hair may fall out. There are many causes of eczema, including allergies, parasites, contact with chemicals, bacterial infections and auto-immune skin diseases.

Diet – Follow the dietary guidelines for allergic pets. Chronic, long-term eczema responds well to fasting, since it helps to cleanse the body of impurities. This can be on a one-day-a-week basis if the condition has been around for some time.

Supplement the diet with kelp tablets or powder, vitamin E (50–300iu daily), zinc (5–20mg daily), vitamin C (500–3,000mg daily), vitamin A (5,000–10,000iu daily), brewer's yeast or a yeast-free B complex daily and oils daily, such as evening primrose oil, fish oil or linseed oil (see chapters three and four).

Environment – Check your pet's environment for allergens, such as moulds, pollens, house dust, house dust mites, fleas or anything that could be causing an allergic reaction. Keep their bed clean and aired.

Aromatherapy – Tea tree and lavender oils can be massaged into the skin. Put a few drops in a base oil like olive oil or sunflower oil and massage straight on to the affected area. Tea tree is antiseptic and soothing and helps to heal sore skin. Lavender is also soothing to the skin. Essential oils can be mixed into a base cream, such as olive oil cream, and used as an ointment on the skin. Some come ready-made as creams for external use.

Bach flower remedies – Crab apple is the cleansing remedy and helps to clear out toxins and bacterial infections. It also helps to rid the animal of unwanted emotions.

Biochemical tissue salts – Use combination D for minor skin complaints, kali. phos. for greasy, scaly skin, kali. sulph. for dry skin, silica for skin that is slow to heal.

Herbs – Use garlic, nettle, aloe vera and valerian. Liquid garlic can be used externally to heal and clean sore skin areas. Garlic taken internally has antiseptic and healing properties and helps to remove internal parasites and fight infection. You can use it raw in your pet's food, or buy ready-made garlic tablets. Nettles are cleansing and purifying and can be used fresh or in tablet form. Aloe vera gel can be spread directly on to the skin and has a soothing and healing effect. Aloe vera is also available as a spray for use on animals. Valerian has a calming effect on the animal's nervous system.

Homoeopathy – Sulphur is the main remedy for skin ailments, especially with redness and warm, itchy skin. Use cantharis for burning, angry skin eruptions, hepar. sulph. for infected, discharging sores on the skin, graphites for eczema with discharge.

Scratching

Scratching can be caused by a number of things, but the two most common triggers are allergies and parasites. A herbal shampoo, such as seaweed and birch, will help to relieve scratching. You could also bathe your pet in water with a few drops of tea tree added. The most important first step, though, is to change your pet's food to a natural allergy-free diet and filtered or bottled water. (Also see eczema and dermatitis and coat problems.)

Smelly animals

A smelly animal is a sure sign that the animal is toxic or is eating an inadequate diet. The smell comes through the skin since this is a major organ of elimination, and when the smell is noticeable it means the body is labouring under a heavy toxic load. Usually poor diet, poor digestion and poor elimination are at the root of this. If your pet has constipation or diarrhoea these need to be addressed as well, along with changing to a natural additive-free diet. If bad breath is a problem, have their teeth and mouth checked out by your vet. Other causes of smelly animals are skin problems, worm infestations and glandular disorders. (Also see constipation, diarrhoea, parasites, skin disorders, anal glands, hormonal problems and ear infections.)

Diet – A change of diet to a natural additive-free regime may be enough to sort the problem out. Many animals will benefit from an occasional day's fast to help them eliminate toxins from the body. Use a good-quality multi-mineral and vitamin supplement for dogs or cats (see chapters three and four).

Bach flower remedies – Use crab apple for cleansing.

Herbs – Aloe vera and garlic are great internal cleansers. Dandelion and nettle help to detox the liver and kidneys.

Homoeopathy – Use nux vomica, given in acute or chronic doses depending on the condition.

Bathing – Both dogs and cats can benefit from being washed. Some cats do not clean themselves properly, which may be the cause of their odour. Pets can be bathed in water with lemon juice or tea tree oil added, or use a natural herbal shampoo.

Exercise – Exercise is also important to help eliminate toxins from the body.

Warts

Warts grow on the skin and are usually harmless. They can grow singly or come in clusters, and often come and go naturally on younger animals who have strong immune systems. Older or weak animals may not naturally get rid of their warts. If a wart gets damaged it can bleed or become infected. It is thought that warts are caused by a virus, and may appear after vaccination.

Diet – Change to a natural preservative-free diet to keep the immune system strong and to lessen the toxic load in the body. Garlic is a great internal cleanser and immune-booster and can be added raw to food. Use a good-quality multi-mineral and vitamin supplement for cats or dogs. Make sure it contains zinc, vitamin C, vitamin A and all the B vitamins. Vitamin E capsules can be opened and dabbed directly on to warts (see chapters three and four).

Aromatherapy – Tea tree or lemon oil can be dabbed on to warts.

Bach flower remedies – Use crab apple for cleansing. Another useful flower remedy for warts is pansy, which is one of the FES and California Research Essences.

Biochemical tissue salts – Use kali. mur. and nat. mur. given together.

Herbs – Use echinacea taken internally to boost the immune system, aloe vera taken internally as a general cleanser. Tree of life can be used topically for treating warts.

Homoeopathy – Thuja is the main remedy for warty growths. You can also dab thuja tincture on to the wart on a daily basis.

SPAYING AND NEUTERING

Whether to spay female pets or neuter male pets comes down to personal choice. However, many unwanted kittens and puppies can be prevented if animals that are free to roam are spayed or neutered. This does require surgery, but there is a lot you can do afterwards to help with the healing process. Neither operation seems to cause long-term health problems, and although the operation can be costly, the PDSA helps those on low incomes by providing free health care for their pets. The best time to have an animal spayed or neutered is once it has reached sexual maturity, assuming you are not going to breed from it.

There are advantages, too. For example, a neutered cat is less likely to roam or spray in the house and often becomes a gentler, less aggressive pet. These operations do not change your pet's personality, and they should not have a problem with weight gain either, unless they are being overfed.

Diet – A good diet and supplement regime will help to speed recovery from the operation. Your pet may also benefit from a short liquid fast immediately after surgery to give its body a chance to heal. Useful additions to the diet to aid recovery include plenty of good-quality protein, garlic, vitamins A, C and E, B complex, zinc, calcium and magnesium (see chapters three and four for advice on diet and supplements). Vitamin E capsules can be opened and rubbed on to operation scars to assist the healing process.

Bach flower remedies – Rescue remedy will help to calm an animal before and after an operation. Clematis helps animals to recover from the anaesthetic. Use crab apple for cleansing after an anaesthetic, olive for an exhausted animal.

Herbs – Comfrey can be taken internally or used externally to promote rapid healing. Comfrey cream can be applied topically on the operation wound. Echinacea taken internally helps to boost the immune system.

Homoeopathy – Use arnica for bruising, aconite immediately before and afterwards for stress and fear. Hypericum helps to relieve pain and repair damaged tissue.

Bibliography

Allport, Richard, BVetMed, VetMFHom, MRCVS, *Heal your Cat the Natural Way*; Mitchell Beazley, 1997.

Allport, Richard, BVetMed, VetMFHom, MRCVS, *Heal your Dog the Natural Way*; Mitchell Beazley, 1997.

Bradford, Nikki, *The Hamlyn Encyclopedia of Complementary Health*; Hamlyn, 1996.

Burton Goldberg Group, The, *Alternative Medicine: The Definitive Guide*; Future Medicine Publishing Inc., 1993.

Clark, Hulda Regehr, *The Cure for all Diseases*; Promotion Publishing, 1995.

Day, Christopher, MA VetMB, MRCVS, VetMFHom, *Homoeopathy: First Aid for Pets*; Chinham Publications, 1992.

Earle, Liz, *Liz Earle's Quick Guides – Aromatherapy*; Boxtree Limited, 1994.

Frazier, Anitra, with Norma Eckroate, *The New Natural Cat*; Plume, 1990.

Grosjean, Nelly, *Veterinary Aromatherapy*; The C.W. Daniel Company Limited, 1994.

Harper, Joan, *The Healthy Cat and Dog Cookbook*; Pet Press, 1975.

Harvey, Clare G. and Amanda Cochrane, *The Encyclopaedia of Flower Remedies*; Thorsons, 1995.

Hunter, Francis, MRCVS, VetMFHom, *Homoeopathic First Aid Treatment for Pets*; Thorsons, 1988.

Lazarus, Pat, *Keep your Pet Healthy the Natural Way*; Keats Publishing Inc., 1986.

McKay, Pat, *Reigning Cats and Dogs*; Oscar Publications, 1992.

MacLeod, George, *Homoeopathy for Pets*; Wigmore Publications Limited, 1981.

Page, Robin, *Animal Cures the Country Way*.

Pitcairn, Richard, DVM, PhD, and Susan Hubble Pitcairn, *Dr Pitcairn's Complete Guide to Natural Health for Dogs and Cats*; Rodale Books, 1995.

Raymonde-Hawkins MBE, M. and George MacLeod, *The Raystede Handbook of Homoeopathic Remedies for Animals*; The C.W. Daniel Company Limited, 1985.

Stanway, Andrew, Dr, *A Guide to Biochemical Tissue Salts*; Van Dyke Books, 1982.

Stein, Diane, *Natural Healing for Dogs and Cats*; The Crossing Press, 1993.

Stein, Diane, *The Natural Remedy Book for Dogs and Cats*; The Crossing Press, 1994.

Vlamis, Gregory, *Rescue Remedy: The Healing Power of Bach Flower Rescue Remedy*; Thorsons, 1994.

Index